BOOK FOR SALE!!!

PRICE: $ 23.00

PLEASE GIVE CHECK OR MONEY TO A.J.

MAKE CHECKS PAYABLE TO:

LISA MARIA FRAGUADA

THANK YOU!

Making
Effective
Referrals

MAKING EFFECTIVE REFERRALS

The Therapeutic Process

By Sharon E. Cheston, Ed.D.

GARDNER PRESS, INC.
NEW YORK LONDON SYDNEY

GARDNER PRESS, INC.
19 Union Square West
New York, New York 10003

Library of Congress Cataloging in Publication Data
Cheston, Sharon E.
Making effective referrals : a therapeutic process / by Sharon E. Cheston.
p. cm.
Includes bibliographical references.
ISBN 0-89876-170-0
1. Psychiatric referral. I. Title.
[DNLM: 1. Counseling. 2. Interpersonal Relations. 3. Psychology, Applied. 4. Referral and Consultation. WM 55 C525m]
RC455.2.R43C48 1990
616.89'14—dc20
DNLM/DLC
for Library of Congress 90-3068
CIP

BOOK DESIGN BY SIDNEY SOLOMON

PRINTED IN THE UNITED STATES OF AMERICA

Preface

The field of counseling and psychotherapy had undergone a predictable maturing process over the last 50 years. As with most human service occupations, the maturing signals an age of specialization. With specialization comes the need to be able to refer clients who do not present problems which are commensurate with one's specialty.

Prior to the movement of specialization, generalists only referred clients with whom they had countertransference issues or who were in need of a totally different type of therapeutic interaction. This activity gave the referral process a negative connotation that still continues today.

If specialization was the result of a maturing process of the mental health field, then a not so positive maturing occurred in the school counseling profession over the last few decades. The profession of school counseling was first conceived to meet the needs of students. However, as the profession suffered fiscal restraint, the profession's counselor/student ratio began to rise and counselors found themselves spending most of their time in career/college guidance, administrative duties, and in crisis intervention. Yet more and more students and their families are presenting serious mental health problems that need attention. Therefore, school counselors find that one of their frequent responsibilities is referral.

Despite the increased need for referral due to specialization among mental health professionals and an increase in counselor/student ratios, the process of referral remains ill-conceived and haphazard. Referral as an activity is not taught routinely in graduate schools and is rarely discussed in the literature. Perhaps reluctance to cover this area of therapy is due to the underlying assumption that graduate schools are in existence to teach students how to work with clients, not how to pass clients on to someone else.

However, counselors and other helpers routinely make referrals. If the referral process is poorly conceived, then the client can feel dismissed, or worse, rejected. These feelings can then precipitate a client's not showing up for the appointment or not following through with the very activity that could help him/her to obtain a mentally healthy functioning. In addition, if referrals are not handled with genuine care and concern for clients' needs, then clients may generalize their negative experiences to view the human service profession as an unhealthy institution that is not in a position to help. Therefore, poor referral practices hurt the entire profession and the clients it is set up to serve.

This book is written as a resource text so that human service practitioners are able to access the various referral topics quickly and receive concrete suggestions for how to handle the various situations that may arise.

The topic of referral has interested me for many years. I noticed that if a person was carefully matched with a counselor who was able to meet his/her therapeutic needs, then there was a better chance that the therapeutic alliance would develop. Thus, taking the additional time to thoughtfully process a referral saved many hours of work later because fewer problems were encountered. In addition, the amount of time and energy necessary to make a thoughtful referral is not much more than what is required to make a poorly conceived referral.

In conclusion, this book was written for the generic human service professional. While the words "counselor" or "therapist" appear frequently in the text, this is more for flow of words than to exclude anyone from benefiting from improved referral techniques. School personnel, lawyers, physicians, and funeral directors (just to name a few) can use the ideas presented to effect a positive referral to mental health professionals and any other human service professionals. Finally, in order to fairly represent both sexes equally and to avoid the tedious "him/her" or "he/she," I have consistently used "he" when referring to the client, "she" when referring to the counselor or therapist, and again "he" when referring to a supervisor. However, in case studies, the gender of each participant is stated and varies from case study to case study.

— *Sharon E. Cheston, Ed.D.*

Contents

DEDICATION

I dedicate this book to my husband, Jim, and my daughters, Shannon and Kelly. Their constant love and support were the impetus to keep going when I wanted to quit.

I further wish to thank my colleagues at Loyola who have assisted my efforts in publishing this book, my many clients who always taught me more than I assisted them, and my supervisees who bravely presented their vulnerabilities and growing edges so that I could gain insight into the referral process.

Above all, I acknowledge that all I am and have is a result of God's grace and I give thanks for the blessings of family, colleagues, supervisees, and clients.

1

The Anatomy of a Referral

DEFINITION OF A REFERRAL

The referral of a client to another helping professional is often a difficult decision because of the many emotional and practical issues that may arise between the counselor and client. The goal of referral is to connect the client, parishioner, or patient with the best possible therapist for the client. However, often referral is viewed as *de*ferral by the therapist because of the therapist's emotional response to having to turn her client over to another professional. The therapist may therefore experience feelings of incompetence, failure, or anger. While referral is the act of therapeutically connecting a client with another helper, deferral is the act of yielding or paying deference to another who is superior or more knowledgeable. The distinction may appear subtle but, in reality, the sense of deferral instead of referral is what intensifies the feelings of guilt, incompetence, and/or rejection when a referral becomes necessary.

While many helpers see the need to refer as an admission of defeat or an admission of their own limitations in working with their clients, the act of referral and the decision to refer is actually an empowering action. The counselor, physician, or minister is in an extremely potent position of recommending the next most appropriate helper for her client. It is through the counselor's community contacts and the accurate assessment of the client's needs that the referral becomes a linkage to the next step toward health for the client.

A referral can sometimes be the most therapeutic intervention that the therapist can make. Whether the referral is being requested by the client or is being initiated by the helper, the act of referral involves separation and grief, and the key act of liaison with the most appropriate referral on the client's behalf.

No matter how difficult the decision to refer is, the only ethical reason to refer is for the well-being of the client. Counselors must think of their clients' needs first, so that the appropriate referral resource is contacted to provide the best possible treatment.

Referral versus Recommendation

Many helpers carry out the act of referral by simply telling their clients that they are not able to continue the counseling relationship and recommending that the client find another counselor. Other counselors will offer clients a list of names of other therapists who may be available to help. These actions do not constitute referral; they are simply recommendations to clients. Referral involves the active participation of both counselor and client in the identification of the client's requirements for a new therapist.

Referral versus Networking

A common mistake that helpers make is confusing the referral of a client with networking with other professionals to provide a wider range of services to the client. Whereas a referral involves the therapist's relinquishing of the primary responsibility for the client's counseling, networking involves the therapist's continuing to be the primary therapeutic agent while coordinating the client's work with other supportive professionals for specific assistance.

Counselors often will hesitate to network with other professionals for fear that clients may become confused by having too many helpers offering assistance, for fear that they may lose control over their clients' counseling, or for fear that the client may be attracted to another helpers work and leave the therapeutic relationship.

Networking During Counseling

Counselors often need to network with other professionals during the counseling relationship. Usually the network referral is for group counseling, medical assistance, specialized individual counseling, or self-help groups.

Group counseling can be a positive adjunct to individual counseling. Group work can provide peer support, peer feedback, socialization skills, and reinforcement to individual counseling. However, group counseling does not provide the intensive one-to-one relationship that can lead to weekly processing of the client's issues. By participating in both individual and group counseling, the client can gain the positive effects of intensive one-to-one interaction as well as peer interaction. Typical presenting issues which are addressed well by conjoint individual and group counseling are: substance abuse, rape, bereavement, adolescent problems, co-dependency, and adult survivors of sexual abuse.

Clients often need medical assistance while in therapy. If the client is seeing a physician, then the counselor needs to work with the physician so that the counseling is effective. If the client is in need of psychiatric or other medical attention, then the counselor networks with medical professionals who can assist the client with his physical problems or drug therapy while continuing counseling.

During family counseling, therapists will sometimes recommend that a family member receive individual counseling. The individual counseling is routinely performed by a therapist other than the family counselor to keep the boundaries clear. Coordination is critical so that the two counselors are not working at odds with each other.

Clients also may need network referral to other types of professionals, such as attorneys, accountants, and funeral directors. It is useful to keep a list of such people. See chapter 6 for additional information on networking.

Case Study: Networking

> Ann entered counseling with a goal of feeling better about herself. She identified three areas in which she needed to see progress in order to gain an increase in her self-esteem. She wanted to lose fifty pounds, to reconnect after twenty years with her alcoholic father, and to learn to accept herself in a noncritical manner. The counselor connected Ann with a local diet center nutritionist who was able to work with Ann behaviorally on her diet and exercise. After working with Ann for a few sessions and noticing her progress with her diet, the counselor assisted Ann in joining an ACoA (Adult Children of Alcoholics) group at her local church. The counselor stayed in touch with Ann about her diet success and the process of her group work while continuing to facilitate Ann's affective and cognitive changes through the weekly therapeutic sessions.

Notice that Ann's counseling was not relinquished to any other professional. Ann is still connected with her counselor and expects that her counselor is coordinating an appropriate network in order to further her progress. To keep this confusion from occurring, counselors need to view themselves as managers.

Managers coordinate the several approaches toward a common goal. Managers, however, do not perform all duties themselves but instead carefully allow the experts to handle their specific areas. As a manager, the counselor will identify when the client needs additional help, will network with the needed expert professionals, but will continue the counseling relationship with the client. Using signed releases of confidential information, the counselor can keep in contact with the expert professional(s) so that the client gets all the help he requires. Therefore, the client recognizes that his counselor is the primary coordinator of his personal growth.

THE REFERRAL PROCESS

The actual procedure of making a referral involves several important steps if the referral is to be a therapeutic experience. First, the decision must be made to refer the client to another helper. Second, contact with the referral source is made to explore whether an effective referral can be made and how it should be worked out. Third, the information must be shared with the client. Finally, the appropriate paperwork completes the process.

The Decision to Refer

Arriving at the decision to refer a client is probably the most emotionally rigorous part of the process. There are numerous reasons to refer, each presenting emotional responses to work through. The reasons to refer that make a decision imminent will be discussed fully in other chapters. The decision to refer is the most time-consuming step in the process of referral and needs to be carefully weighed by the counselor. It is during this stage that the counselor needs to rely on supervision or consultation with a colleague. Once the decision to refer is made, the counselor must decide upon the appropriate referral resource. The match between the referral resource and the client is particularly critical to the success of the relationship-building potential. Research shows that the relationship between the professional helper and the client is the most significant predictor of counseling success. Therefore, it is crucial to consider whether or not there is the potential for a therapeutic relationship between the client who is being referred and the referral resource.

In order to assist the counselor in determining whether the referral resource being considered is the most appropriate helper, several questions can be asked:

- Are the client and referral resource intellectually compatible?
- Are the client and referral resource emotionally compatible?
- Are they spiritually compatible?

- Is there a compatibility involving physical location, affordability, and accessibility?
- Does the referral resource have the requisite credentials to assist this client?
- If this is a cross-cultural referral, does the therapist possess the skills and sensitivity to assist someone of the client's race or culture?
- If this referral is cross-sexual, is this fact going to be therapeutic for the client or might it stand in the way of his growth?

By pondering the answers to these questions for each referral resource, the referring therapist can make a potentially effective referral for her client.

Contact with the Prospective Referral Resources

When a referral is being considered, many professionals question what type of information can and should be shared with the referral resource. A counselor might share too little information for fear of breaching confidentiality of for fear of prejudicing the referral resource. On the other hand, a counselor might share too much information hoping to convince the referral resource to take the client or to convince the referral resource of the counselor's competence in working with the client.

How much information to share depends on whether the counselor contacts the referral resource before or after having discussed the referral with the client. If the counselor has not discussed the referral with the client, then it is prudent to share as little as possible concerning the identification of the client. However, the therapist can explore several areas:

1. Is the referral resource receiving referrals at present? This inquiry is extremely important because the counselor will probably not want her client to be placed on a waiting list.

2. Would the referral resource feel comfortable seeing a client with a presenting problem similar to the client's problem? The

therapist can share the general elements of the client's presenting problems without specifying who the client is.

3. How should the referral be handled? That is, would the referral resource wish to have the client call her, or would the referral resource prefer to call the client?

If the therapist has already discussed the referral with the client and has received permission to explore the referral possibilities, then the client can sign a release of confidential information allowing the counselor the freedom to contact referral resources. The therapist is now free to share knowledge and impressions of the client with the referral resources. If the helper is a clergy person and not comfortable or familiar with having parishioners sign releases, then she should consider beginning this practice. Parishioners may feel even more comfortable if they know that their pastor takes confidentiality seriously and would not talk to another helper with written consent. If the pastor is still uncomfortable with the practice of signed releases for parishioners, then the most appropriate referral stance may be to give the parishioner a list of trusted referral resources who match the parishioner's needs and leave it to the client's own initiative to contact the resources. However, most clergy find that their parishioners are more apt to follow through if personal contact is made by their pastor with the referral resource.

If the helper is calling several resources to test their receptively to a referral, it is best to keep the identification of the client, patient, or parishioner confidential until she has decided to whom she will refer. This practice is wise even if signed releases of confidential information have been obtained.

If the therapist's policy is to give the client three referral possibilities and let the client decide whom he will contact, then the counselor can contact the three referral resources and let them know that they may be receiving a contact from one of the counselor's clients and the type of presenting problem the client has identified. The counselor should also instruct the client to mention her name during the initial contact. This practice builds networks and reciprocity with referral resources.

Sharing Referral Information with Clients

Clients need concrete information, time to process the referral, and support through the process. These subjects are covered thoroughly in other chapters of this book.

Completing the Paperwork

In the helping professions, there is no standardized paperwork that assists a counselor in processing a referral. However, there are several areas that are professionally well served if accompanied by germane referral paperwork.

1. *Release of Confidential Information.* Although completing a release of confidential information is not obligatory in order for a helping professional to speak to a referral resource about an unidentified prospective client, obtaining a release and sending a copy to the referral resources allows the referral information to flow between the two helpers as long as the client permits. The release also formalizes the referral and permits the helpers the freedom to talk honestly and openly because of the executed document. A sample release is shown in Appendix A.

2. *Referral Information Form.* The referral information form lists the information that the client will need to follow up on the referral resources. Clients will follow through on a written referral quicker than they will on a verbal referral. The referral information form lists all referral resources that are being suggested, and their addresses and telephone numbers. The therapist can even draw maps on the back of the form to assist the client in finding the referral resources' offices. An example of this type of form is also shown in Appendix A.

3. *Network Lists.* It is also useful to compile a list of all the services, agencies, and organizations that deal with specific problems which clients can access in their geographical area. Such a list might include AA meetings, Co-dependency or ACoA groups, teen suicide support groups, or compassionate friends. The agency's or practice's logo, name, address, and telephone numbers should be a

part of each network list because the list is also a useful marketing tool.

ASSESSING WHEN REFERRAL IS IN ORDER

There are as many reasons for a counselor to make a referral as there are people who need referral. However, there are categories of reasons for referral:

1. The counselor feels her skill levels are not strong enough to handle the client's needs.
2. The counselor's countertransference is interfering with the therapeutic alliance.
3. The client's resistance seems to be directed at the counselor with no apparent resolution.
4. The counselor is leaving the area.
5. The client is leaving the area.
6. The client is ready to deal with an area requiring a specialist.
7. The client-counselor "fit" is not working.
8. The potential client is a family member or friend.

A pastor who is performing counseling in her own parish may refer a parishioner for all of the above reasons, but, in addition, a pastor may also need to refer a parishioner with whom the pastor works closely in the parish. The pastor may feel that there is a conflict of interest in working with the parishioner both as a client and as a parish worker.

CLIENTS' NEED FOR REFERRAL

Clients may need to be referred to another counselor for several reasons. Clients may need a counselor with a different theoretical approach. For example, if the counselor is primarily behaviorally oriented and the client is struggling with spiritual issues, the referral may need to be made to a pastoral counselor. If the counselor is theoretically person-centered and the client is attempting to overcome a phobia, perhaps the counselor should refer to a behaviorally oriented counselor.

A client may need to be referred because the client and counselor are not developing a working therapeutic relationship. The lack of a relationship may have very little to do with the therapist. For example, there may be transference from the client to the counselor that may be a result of the client's previous experience. The client may be unable to work through this transference presently with this therapist. Referral to another counselor can often assist in giving the client space to work through the current transference issue with another counselor. For example, a client can sometimes be more effectively helped by a therapist of one sex than another, or a client may need a therapist who is older, or younger, or a client may need a counselor of his own race because of the shared cultural experience.

Case Study: Referral for Specialty Counseling

> Sara was referred to a female counselor by a male counselor because Sara had revealed to him that she has been sexually abused as a child but could not bring herself to discuss the incidents with a male at this time. Sara had an excellent relationship with her male counselor but could not discuss this one problem with him. Sara's counselor referred her to a female counselor who focused on Sara's need to discuss the abuse and to integrate the events into her self-concept. Once Sara was more comfortable with her past, she desired marriage counseling and decided to return to her male counselor with her husband because the male counselor was of the same race and religion as she and her husband.

Clients may feel the need to be referred but may not feel the freedom to express their need for fear of being disloyal to their relationship with their counselor. At this point, clients will sometimes discuss termination, which they view as the normal process, rather than bring up the subject of referral. Counselors who are sensitive to the unfinished business of their clients can assist their clients in considering referral rather than termination. If referral occurs rather than termination, then the counselor can continue to be therapeutic by:

1. Modeling letting go and grieving over ending a close relationship;
2. Modeling openness in dealing with the need to seek additional help without becoming defensive;
3. Assisting the client in contacting a new therapist who is a competent professional;
4. Assisting the client in getting additional help rather than terminating, which might mean that the client would not receive the counseling that he needs.

COUNSELORS' NEED FOR REFERRAL

The usual reason for a counselor to consider referral is irreconcilable countertransference toward the client. Counselors often have strong feelings for their clients because the client-counselor relationship is an intense, intimate one. Counselors attempt to hide their feelings from the client, but a more therapeutic approach is for the counselor honestly to evaluate her feelings, and to own her affect. If these feelings get in the way of the therapeutic relationship, then referral is in order. Sometimes a counselor will enter counseling herself to work through the countertransference. However, attention must also be paid to the client's needs. If a counselor is unable to quickly identify and work through the countertransference, then referral of the client would be critical.

Another reason a counselor may need to refer is if she is at an impasse in her ability to assist the client. This recognition is a very difficult one for the counselor and can cause feelings of incompetence, depression, failure, and/or guilt. Working with these feelings is discussed more thoroughly later in this book.

Finally, there are more practical needs that call for referral, such as relocation or illness. While these reasons for referral may not evoke the feelings of failure or incompetence, they still indicate that some client and counselor grieving is necessary and still require appropriate referral practices.

Counselors need to be in touch with their own personal issues so that when countertransference occurs, they are open to viewing their vulnerabilities. Also, by staying in touch with their own issues and by being open to exploring them, counselors will recognize more quickly when countertransference occurs.

Some counselors have problems dealing with the recognition that a client is not making progress because of their inability to deal with him and his issues. A counselor may use denial to protect herself from the painful fact that she cannot help her client. To face a shortcoming is to admit one's own limitations and humans do not like to own limitations. Feelings of inadequacy can overwhelm a counselor and spur her to work harder, becoming even more determined to succeed. This postpones the client receiving the help he needs and also may cause the client to cease working while the counselor is working on her own therapeutic issues. Finally, some counselors find it easier to blame the client for the lack of progress than to face their own vulnerabilities. Counselors will sometimes call the client resistant, well-defended, and out of touch with his feelings, rather than explore their own role in the therapeutic relationship.

Supervision, or at least collegial sharing, can alert counselors to times when their skills, relationships, or personal assets are limiting their clients' growth.

WHY COUNSELORS AND OTHERS DO NOT REFER

Counselors often are reluctant to refer their clients and cite the following reasons:

1. Loss of income;
2. Lack of referral resources in their area;

3. Belief that no other counselor could work any more effectively with the difficult client;
4. Fear that the client will feel rejected;
5. Fear of loss of credibility with the referred client or with colleagues.

In addition, some ministers who do counseling in their parish will say that they do not wish to refer to a secular counselor, psychologist, or psychiatrist because they feel that their client's (parishioner's) religious faith will not be understood or respected. Ministers report that they will keep working with a client in hopes that they can reach him through their relationship even though they feel less than competent to deal with the client's issues. (See Chapter 13)

1. *Loss of Income.* While losing a client often means a temporary loss of income, this reason alone must never impede the process of a client's receiving the best help possible. While counselors and other helpers are not called upon to take a professional oath, such as physicians are, it is critical that counselors embrace their profession as a dedication to helping others. Counselors must never further their own finances at the expense of the client's mental health.

2. *Lack of Referral Resources.* The lack of referral resources can be a problem for counselors working in isolated small communities or rural areas. However, recently three counselors from West Virginia reported that their answer to the problem of isolation and lack of community resources was to seek out each other, identify together their personal, professional, and community resources, and then to establish their own limited referral group. As they sought each other out, they also found a nurse, a physician, a minister, and a state worker who shared their problem of isolation and were willing to pool their knowledge of resources. In this situation, counselors need to broaden their concept of "therapy." Professional counselors, social workers, psychiatric nurses, psychologists, psychiatrists, pastoral counselors, and ministers are all in the business of helping people, and looking beyond one's own professional circles can bring enhancement of known resources.

3. *Feeling That No Other Counselor Could Work More Effectively*

with the Client. A counselor can believe that her client is so well-defended or resistant that no one could effect any change in him. While this is true in some cases, the counselor needs to explore whether this is really true or whether the client could benefit from referral. Being honest with one's feelings and thoughts may open the door to a referral and, therefore, to a more therapeutic relationship for the client.

4. *Client's Feeling of Rejection.* Clients are seen as people who cannot stand rejection and referral is seen by many counselors as rejection. Referring a client by matching the best suited therapist with the client is not rejection. In fact, it is affirmation that the counselor cares for her client and wants the best help available for him.

5. *Loss of Face with Client and Colleagues.* A counselor who assumes that a referral means loss of face with her client or referral colleague may be hesitant to refer. Clients appreciate honest communication, especially when their best interest is involved, and usually will respect the counselor more for an appropriate referral than for allowing the client to keep coming when more appropriate help is available elsewhere. Colleagues, too, admire openness and honesty in their fellow therapists and would respect a therapist who has the integrity to refer in a difficult situation rather than digging in her heels and preventing the client from getting the help he needs.

TYPES OF NONTHERAPEUTIC REFERRAL

Referrals that are therapeutic are well thought out, caring, sensitive to the needs of the client. However, according to Miach, Elliott, and Cava (1979) many professionals refer clients with a hidden agenda. They have placed these nontherapeutic referral into six categories:

1. *Magical-Expectations Referral.* This type of referral occurs when the client has unreasonable expectations about the outcome of the therapy which the helper has failed to recognize as unreasonable. Realizing she is unable to meet the client's expectations, the

counselor refers the client to another therapist or institution. However, the expectations of the client are "magical" and cannot be fulfilled by anyone. The failure to recognize the client's expression of wants as magical expectations will lead to disappointment on the part of both client and counselor. Counselors need to be able to assess clients' expectations of counseling with a critical eye so they can make realistic appraisals of the validity of their expectations.

2. *Prescriptive Referral.* A referral of this sort occurs when a counselor refers a client to another professional helper and then proceeds to instruct the helper as to how to handle the client. The most common form of prescriptive referral is often covert and implicit in the supervisory relationship where the supervisor refers a client to the supervisee and then proceeds to tell the supervisee how to work with the client. However, referring counselors can have trouble relinquishing a client to another, and so refer but then impose their opinions as to how the therapy should progress onto the new counselor.

3. *Disavowed Consultation.* When a client becomes frustrated or resistant with his counselor and refers himself to another counselor, a clash can occur if the original counselor is not receptive to the referral. The manipulation by the client needs to be assessed by the new therapist and it is recommended that the new therapist refuse to see the client until he returns to his original counselor and terminates the relationship. In this way, the previous therapeutic relationships clearly ended before another one is begun. Also, this process will keep the client from running away from therapy without the counselor's having a chance to confront the client's flight or resistance and enabling a therapeutic referral.

4. *Slough Referral.* A slough referral occurs when a referring counselor wishes to get the client off her hands so she refers the client to another or uses in-patient admission as the referral. There is nothing wrong with referring a client if the counselor does not feel she can work with the client any longer. However, a slough referral is referring without thought or consideration of the client's needs. One client recognized a slough referral when she said to her counselor, "The only reason that you hospitalized me was so that you could sleep well at night knowing I was safe." The counselor

admitted in supervision that this thought had been one motivation for the hospitalization.

5. *Disguised Crisis Intervention.* When a client wishes a referral, he can fabricate a crisis that requires hospitalization or a different therapeutic intervention. However after the referral, the crisis quickly dissipates. When the crisis first occurs, the referring therapist is often unable to discern it as a disguised wish for referral. The new therapist will be able to assess the transitory crisis and watch for the pattern to be repeated, so that the client's behavior can be confronted the next time.

6. *Inverse Referral.* An inverse referral occurs when a client is referred for reasons about which the referring counselor is unclear. She may have been coaxed into the referral by the client or may just let go without a struggle or a question.

These referral types should be avoided for they are counterproductive to the therapeutic process.

CONCLUSION

Referral is a process which has commonly been seen as an admission of failure of the therapeutic process. However, the basic premise of referral is the connection of a client with the most appropriate helping resource available. Keeping this basic premise in focus rather than concentrating on negative feelings will assist helpers to view referral as a therapeutic process.

2

Locating, Developing, Maintaining, and Evaluating Referral Resources

Referral resources are readily available in cities and towns across the country. However, counselors need to know not only how to find resources but also how to evaluate and maintain these resources.

LOCATING REFERRAL RESOURCES

Below, there are several suggestions as to where to look for resources.

1. *Professional Colleagues.* The most obvious place to start searching for referral resources is the collegial environment in which the counselor normally operates. Colleagues are natural resources because the counselor frequently interacts with professional colleagues and is often familiar with the type and quality of work of her colleagues. Also, because communication is so frequent, maintaining the resource is easy.

2. *Colleagues of Colleagues.* When a counselor is in need of a

specialist, one place to start is to pick the brain of a colleague. Professional colleagues can be valuable proveniences of referral resources. One professional can often know someone who knows someone.

When a counselor uses resources suggested by a colleague which she has not had the opportunity to research herself, she must rely on her colleague's knowledge and judgment. In order to make this process most effective, the counselor should carefully describe to her colleague exactly what her specific referral needs are, and then follow up the referral with a thorough evaluation of its outcome.

3. *Local Universities.* Local or regional colleges and universities which have psychology, counseling, community mental health, or social work departments employ teachers who teach courses in the helping professions. In addition to their own private practices, teachers are often well connected to the professional community including other universities, professional organizations, and counseling agencies. Teachers may also have connections to the alumni or alumnae who practice counseling or therapy in the counselor's area.

4. *Professional Organization.* As a professional helper, a therapist needs to connect with the professional organizations in her field. Activity in professional organizations will assist a therapist not only with professional identity but also with referral resources. Membership lists are rich sources of referrals. Conventions and meetings are excellent places to make contacts with other professionals who may be possible referral resources.

5. *Continuing Education Workshops.* Attendance at workshops and professional seminars can assist counselors in learning about new advances in the field as well as in networking with other professionals who can develop into referral resources.

6. *The Telephone Book.* The phone book can serve as a beginning list of resources for those therapists who are totally new to an area. However, extreme caution must be exercised in randomly drawing a referral resource from the phone book because there is no ready means by which to evaluate the helpers listed in the Yellow Pages. Many reputable therapists advertise in the Yellow Pages and may become valuable resources for the therapist. On the other

hand, there are many untrained people in practice who also utilize the Yellow Pages to advertise. The telephone book publishers do not assess credentials before taking an order for an ad. One way to begin the evaluation process is to write to the therapists and agencies listed in the phone book asking for their cards, brochures, and/or catalogs. From this information, the counselor can ascertain credentials and decide whether the prospective referral resource has the background that the counselor is seeking.

7. *The Local Community.* Finally, keep in mind that there are a myriad of opportunities for locating referral resources in the community. Friends, neighbors, business contacts, and social acquaintances can provide leads to resources. Being continually alert for opportunities to encounter new referral resources will also assist the counselor in developing a steady influx of referrals for her own practice.

BUILDING REFERRAL RESOURCES LISTS

Once the therapist knows the types of referrals she is apt to need to make, it is advisable to make detailed lists, a directory, or a business card file of the referral resources that are most frequently needed. Among the resources that a therapist typically needs are psychiatrists, psychologists, mental health counselors, drug and alcohol abuse counselors, pastoral counselors, rehabilitation counselors, career and guidance counselors, Alcoholics Anonymous meetings, Gamblers Anonymous meeting, eating disorders clinics, Overeaters Anonymous meetings, mental health clinics, suicide prevention teams, mental hospitals, and Adult Children of Alcoholics (co-dependency) groups. These referral resources seem to surface over and over again as therapists work with clients, but they are only a starting point. Most therapists find that as they work in the field their lists grow more extensive.

It is wise to research the appropriateness and efficacy of the referral resources before being faced with the need to make a referral. Prior planning prevents hasty, poorly conceived referrals.

Instead of trying to build a complete referral list all at once, the therapist should develop one of two reliable referral resources in each category and then build on those as her professional circles develop and expand.

DEVELOPING REFERRAL RESOURCES

Cultivating a wide variety of referral resources aids the counselor in connecting her client with the most therapeutic relationship possible. However, there is another benefit to developing referral resources. The counselor in turn becomes a referral resource for those she is cultivating for her own list. This type of collegial interface benfits both parties. Therefore, counselors should not hesitate to make the necessary contacts with other professionals to obtain referral resources and to become a resource herself.

Making Contact

Often, counselors fear that contacting another helper for the purpose of referral may place them in an inferior or needy position vis à vis the referral resource. Building a stronger network of referral resources does not make one inferior to other helpers. Quite the contrary, the more networks to which one is connected and the more professionals one knows, the more empowered one becomes as a therapist. The well-connected therapist is empowered not only by her access to a large list of referral resources and participation in many professional circles, but also by her growing reputation as an excellent resource herself. Her referrals to others will be well-thought-out and appropriate to each client's needs, while at the same time her own professional opportunities will be enhanced.

There are basically two ways to make the initial contact with another professional: written and oral. If the contact is written, the communiqué is often tossed away before the recipient reads even a couple of lines because *so* much information comes across professional desks. The oral means has its problems too. The greatest obstacle to overcome in the cold call is the possible rejection that may occur.

A counselor can try a combination of approaches by first sending a written note stating that she will be following up with a phone call later. This can work well, but there is still the possibility of rejection or misunderstanding. The person contacted may interpret the overture as an attempt to obtain client referrals, rather than to identify referral resources. If the contact has this perception, then the counselor will be seen as a threat rather than as a colleague. One possible way to overcome this concern is to have a referral in mind when the call is placed to show the referral intention. If this is impossible, then the alternative is to listen carefully to what is being said and to what is not being said and affirm the desire to develop professional resources that are of a collegial nature. If the prospective referral resource still seems to feel threatened or reluctant to meet, then that referral resource is probably not one that would yield positive results.

The best means of making contact with a new referral resource is through a mutual professional colleague or friend whom the counselor already knows and respects. The mutual colleague can make the initial contact for the counselor, alerting the prospective referral resource of the counselor's strengths and good will and of the counselor's intention to make a contact. This method of contact reduces the possibility of rejection and of the counselor being seen as a possible threat.

The Followup Meeting

When meeting with the prospective referral resource, the counselor can facilitate the meeting by asking a few clarifying questions. First, to get an idea of the referral resource's areas of expertise, the counselor can ask him to list the types of presenting problems that he feels he handles best as a professional. Second, the counselor can ask about the background and credentials of the referral resource. These questions need not be threatening or cause evasiveness.

Simple straightforward questions can be seen as interest on the part of the counselor. Some typical questions that may help the conversation could include:

- What did you do before you entered private practice (or your present agency)?
- What areas of work do you enjoy the most?
- With which types of clients do you feel the most competent?
- Do you offer any workshops or group sessions?

The counselor can react to the responses to her questions and then end the meeting by asking how the new referral resource prefers to receive referrals. Some referral resources prefer that the referring counselor contact them with the name and phone number of the client and then the referral resource makes the contact. Still others prefer that the counselor do both. That is, the counselor gives the referral resource the client's name and phone number and gives the client the referral resource's name and phone number. Whichever way the new referral resource prefers referrals to be handled, it is crucial for the counselor to know this information and respect the requested procedure.

Finally, the counselor makes a referral to the referral resource or, if no immediate referral is in the offing, sends a follow-up note thanking the referral resource for his time and professional information.

MAINTAINING REFERRAL RESOURCES

Occasionally, long periods of time may pass without the helper needing to make referrals and, therefore, the frequent contact once enjoyed by the helper and the referral resource seems to dwindle or even cease. During these times it is important not to let the referral resources forget the counselor, both to maintain the referral relationships so that referrals can be handled expediently in the future and to prevent the possibility of reciprocal referrals from fading.

There are several means by which to maintain the valuable referral resources which have been cultivated.

1. Call the referral resources periodically to update the file and to let them know that they are still a part of the resource file.
2. Seek out the referral resources at meetings, conventions, and other gatherings to reinforce your presence to them.
3. Send announcements of groups, workshops, speeches and/or changes to the practice; for example, adding a staff member or relocating.
4. Send thank you notes to any referral resource who refers a client to you.
5. Send thank you notes to any referral resource who accepts a referral from you.
6. Send out new brochures with personal notes to each resource.
7. Prepare newsletters and send them to referral resources, and to clients, colleagues, friends, and neighbors as well.
8. Keep personal information in a referral resource file such as birthday, anniversary, and special events and send cards on these days with personal notes.
9. Keep a supply of sympathy, congratulations, and get-well cards and send them to the referral resources whenever they are ill, experiencing grief, or enjoying success.

FINDING REFERRAL RESOURCES THROUGH NETWORKING

Networking helps to build a referral resource base, but is not the resource base itself. Networking can be accomplished through many people who would not necessarily qualify as a referral resource. For example, at a social gathering the counselor may talk to a funeral director in her town. The funeral director would seldom receive referrals from the counselor but could act as a valuable network link to other professionals who may develop into referral resources and, in addition, may visualize the counselor as a potential referral resource.

One way of establishing network links is to carry business cards at all times and when a network possibility presents itself, jot a note on the back of a business card and hand it to the possible link. Later, a follow-up phone call can begin the process of networking to and through this new acquaintance.

The important idea for a counselor to remember is that professionals outside the helping professions often have contacts with practitioners in the helping professions. These contacts can assist the counselor in networking with other professionals, can act as referral sources to the counselor, and can assist the counselor in marketing her practice. The point is not to neglect the large segment of the population that is business- or service-oriented.

EVALUATING REFERRAL RESOURCES

After the referral resource has been established and cultivated, and a referral has been made, the counselor must evaluate how well the referral relationship is functioning.

Therapists want to ascertain how the referral process has progressed from both the resource's point of view and the client's, whether the client feels appropriately connected to his new helper, and how the referral procedure could be improved. Essentially, the counselor needs to know whether or not she can confidently use the same referral resource and referral process again.

Frequently, the counselor will receive feedback spontaneously when the client is happy or unhappy with the referral. Obviously, the counselor needs to take into consideration the client's pathology when receiving the client's evaluation. A client could complain even when the referral resource is exactly the type of help the client needs because he does not want that help. However, it is appropriate to listen to the referred client because he is a consumer of services, and your reputation, as well as that of the referral resource, is at stake if the referral goes awry.

To evaluate a new referral resource, the counselor can contact the referral resource a few weeks after the referral and ask how the referral progressed from the resource's perspective. This call will also help to confirm whether the client followed through. If all appears well from the resource's point of view, then a note to the client affirming the new relationship can assist the client in knowing that the counselor is concerned with his welfare. If the client is unhappy, the note can motivate a phone call to the counselor.

If the client did not follow through with the referral, then the referral resource may be able to explain how the process broke down. In this instance, the referring counselor can call the client and express concern over the referral *process* and whether the counselor can assist with another referral. If there was a problem with the referral resource, the problem will probably emerge at this time and will give the counselor a chance to evaluate the referral resource as well as the referral process.

Case Study: Referring Counselor's Followthrough

Anna is a thirty-two-year-old white married female who presented herself for counseling because of a feeling of self-hatred. The counselor's practice was full at the time and rather than placing Anna on a waiting list, the counselor decided to refer because of the intensity of Anna's feeling and possible suicidal ideation.

Prior to Anna's contact with the counselor, the counselor had an initial meeting with a new referral resource who presented himself as a dynamic, cognitively oriented counselor who engaged clients quickly and bonded will. Two other colleagues had enthusiastically endorsed this new referral resource. The counselor referred Anna to the new resource.

After one month, the counselor called the new referral resource and found out that Anna had made contact, attended four sessions, and then canceled her appointments. The resource could offer no explanation as to why Anna canceled except that he felt Anna was well-defended and not ready for

> the necessary changes she would have to make. The counselor called Anna, who was very grateful that the counselor had cared enough to call.
>
> Anna reported that the referral resource had shown up late two of the four times she had seen him, had forgotten one appointment, and when they did meet had said nothing, just sat and nodded. Anna was discouraged but agreed to see someone else whom the counselor recommended. This time the counselor used a referral resource which had been consistently successful in the past. Anna saw the new therapist, bonded well, and was very appreciative of the counselor's followthrough.

The feedback received by the counselor in the above scenario was very valuable. It was important to hear both sides of the relationship problem before deciding on a course of action. Clients and referral resources do not always bond well even if the client is well-motivated and the counselor is well-recommended.

The amount of effort that the counselor expended in the above case study may seem excessive but, in fact, required only two phone calls and probably no more than fifteen minutes. The rewards in taking the time to follow up with this referral were: (1) The client felt affirmed, which was a therapeutic issue for her; (2) The counselor received feedback on one of her referral resources'; (3) Six months later, the client referred two more clients to the counselor because of the care and concern with which she handled the referral; and (4) The client did not feel rejected even though she had been referred.

3

Assessing When the Time Is Right for Referral

REFERRAL THAT OCCURS BEFORE THE COUNSELING RELATIONSHIP BEGINS

When the Counselor Is Unable to Take on a Client

Sometimes when a prospective client contacts a counselor, she may be unable to take on a new client. The counselor may not be able to arrive at a convenient time frame with the client, may be at the upper limit of her client load, or may be going on a holiday. Whatever the reason when this occurs, the counselor and the prospective client need to decide whether the client can be placed on the counselor's wait list or be referred to another counselor either immediately or right after an intake interview. Research on wait lists is presented in other sections of this book; this chapter will consider decisions to refer.

There are many considerations to be weighed when making the decision to wait-list or refer. One issue to be assessed is the degree of crisis the client is experiencing. If the client is in the middle of a crisis, then the counselor needs to refer to a counselor who can respond immediately. Another reason to refer rather than to wait-list is if the counselor determines that the client has had unresolved problems for many years but is presently motivated to address the necessary issues. Referral to a counselor who can begin working with the client immediately is more appropriate than placing the client on a wait list where the time lag may cause motivation to wane.

However, it is important to be aware that clients can sometimes be quite resistant to referral once they have taken the risk of making the initial contact with the counselor. For example, a client may de-intensify a crisis or devalue his problem when the counselor recommends that a referral will meet his needs better than being placed on a waiting list. One way to overcome resistance is to work with the prospective client to help him understand that he is entitled to timely assistance with the best helper *available.*

Even if a client is not presenting a crisis or emergency that needs attention, the client often has had to build up courage over weeks to make the initial contact. The counselor needs to be sensitive to this courage and take advantage of the moment before the client loses his commitment. Postponing the client through wait-listing may cause the client to reconsider and not follow through. Counselors often object that if timely intervention is crucial to a client's motivation, then the client is really not motivated to change. However, researchers have demonstrated that the relationship between the counselor and client is the most important determinant of counseling success. An effective, timely, therapeutic referral can take advantage of the client's state of need and motivation. Postponing counseling may lead to the client's losing motivation and not following through with the therapeutic relationship.

What frequently happens is this: the client wonders whether he needs help, waits and monitors himself and his problem for a period of time, seeks a referral name from a trusted source, builds up courage, and then decides to make contact with a counselor. If that contact does not begin a positive process that leads to a relationship, then the client may begin to question his decision. This questioning may lead to a decision not to follow through at this time. Clients are looking for any excuse to change their minds. One client summed it up, "I have to know that the time, emotional energy, and money is going to be worth it. When I had a bad experience of being placed on a waiting list for two months, I questioned whether this was going to be worth it and then didn't follow through for a year. By that time, I was in crisis."

When the Presenting Problem is Beyond the Scope of the Counselor's Skills

Another occasion when a client may be referred before any counseling sessions occur is when the counselor recognizes immediately that the client's presenting problem is incompatible with her own skills or comfort level. Shakespeare admonishes in *Hamlet* "to thine own self be true." It is imperative for helpers to know themselves well, their assets and growing edges. When counselors are able to distinguish between types of clients they are able to work with and those with which they are unlikely to succeed, they are able to be more helpful to their clients, both in actual counseling and in knowing when to make a referral. In turn, referring counselors are able to make more appropriate referral decisions when they know their referral resources know their own strengths and weaknesses. In clinical situations, supervisors who have the freedom to take counselor skill level, interest area, assets, and growing into consideration when client assignment is made, can make more appropriate counselor/client linkages. Whenever a counselor comes into contact with a client who is presenting problems that are outside her skill level, is hooking the counselor's countertransference issues, or is presenting problems that are not within the counselor's interests, then the counselor needs to refer the client to another counselor whose interests, skills, and issues are more compatible.

For a variety of reasons, this effective referral process does not always happen. For example, financial considerations sometimes obscure the goal of therapy. When a client presents himself as being able and willing to pay for the counselor's services, the counselor is tempted to not refer even when referral would be more appropriate. This becomes an ethical and legal question when lack of skills and countertransference issues are involved. These ethical and legal issues will be discussed more thoroughly later in the book. It is critical to keep counseling's basic premise always in sight: Counseling is to help the client in the most therapeutic manner possible. When counselors keep clients who would be better served by a more experienced or differently trained counselor or one who does not have the same countertransference issues, then the basic premise of counseling is violated.

When there are questionable gray areas, supervision is very helpful. A client can be retained even when the counselor feels inexperienced if the counselor has a supervisor who is able to give immediate and on-going critique of her work. If a counselor knows herself well and is receiving supervision, then together the counselor and supervisor can ascertain whether the client's problem is truly beyond the counselor's skill level at this time, or whether with proper supervision the counselor can retain the client and learn from the experience.

Case Study: Referral Due to Inexperience of Counselor

> Carol graduated with a master's degree in counseling, had had one year of counseling experience, and was receiving supervision weekly. A local minister referred a woman named Sheila to Carol because he felt that Sheila needed a female counselor. When Carol asked the minister why Sheila needed counseling, she was told that Sheila had been married three times, had been in and out of relationships with a dozen men, and had tried to commit suicide three times. The minister believed that Sheila did not really want to die but was just trying to get attention. The minister also told Carol of Sheila's sexual abuse as a child and concluded that Sheila could benefit from a female counselor because of the abuse and her unstable relationships with men. Carol felt totally overwhelmed. This was the first referral she had received from this minister and she was afraid that if she referred Sheila, then her referral resource would be disappointed in her ability to handle clients. Carol

called Sheila and talked briefly with her on the phone but after talking with Sheila, Carol felt even more overwhelmed than ever. Carol talked with her supervisor and together they agreed that Sheila would best be treated by a therapist skilled in working with personality disorders, especially borderlines. However, for Carol, the difficult task was communicating the information both to Sheila and to the minister who had referred her. Carol's supervisor suggested that she approach both with the attitude of professional concern that the client receive the best help available. Carol called the minister, told him that after carefully considering Sheila's needs, she was going to refer her to a specialist in women survivors of incest and personality disorders. To Carol's surprise the minister was relieved and grateful that Carol had taken time to listen, to make a tentative diagnosis, and to refer Sheila to an appropriate therapist. Carol's contact with Sheila did not go quite as well. In fact, Sheila suspected that Carol was not feeling skilled enough to handle her problem. Carol, however, maintained her professional stance of concern for Sheila and finally Sheila agreed to see the new counselor.

In this case, Carol was not ready to enter into a therapeutic relationship with a client who was presenting problems such as Sheila was. This incident occurred in 1978. In 1981, Carol received a referral of a similar client and accepted her tentatively while utilizing weekly supervision. After three years of experience, Carol felt that she had acquired many skills and much knowledge which allowed her to build the confidence she needed to take on the difficult problems of a client with a borderline personality disorder. Through supervision, Carol grew in her therapeutic skills and by 1986 Carol became the referral resource for other therapists who needed to refer clients with personality disorders.

Carol's growth as a therapist points out that although we may feel incapable of handling a difficult client at one time, it does not mean that we are never going to be capable of handling a difficult client. Also important is the fact that Carol's relationship with the minister was not destroyed because of her inability to handle Sheila's problems.

When the Client Is a Family Member, Friend, or Friend of the Family

The final reason for a client to be referred before the counseling relationship begins is when friends and family request counseling. As a helper, you will encounter many family members and friends who will feel free to approach you for your expertise. Although helpers are aware of the ethical taboos against counseling family members and friends, there are many gray areas that can cause the counselor to feel uncomfortable. For example, should a counselor work directly with the friend of the counselor's child or spouse? Some counselors feel that friends of immediate family members are acceptable as clients as long as the counselor is not a friend of the prospective client as well. However, other counselors believe that friends of family members are too close to the therapist for clear boundaries to be retained in the therapeutic relationship. In such cases the counselor should ask herself if, when the therapeutic relationship undergoes difficult times, the client would have the power to cause a strain between the counselor and a family member or significant other. If the answer to the question is yes, then the client should be referred.

Case Study: Referral due to Conflict of Interest

> A counselor named Erin was working with her daughter's school friend, Kim. Erin did not know Kim before they started therapy, but Erin's daughter knew and socialized with Kim. During the therapy, Erin was called upon to confront Kim with her self-defeating behavior. Kim experienced anger and began talking to Erin's daughter about how Erin was counseling her. Erin's daughter was caught in a difficult position and although she tried to stay out of Erin's and Kim's relationship, Kim tried to use Erin's daughter to manipulate Erin. Erin found that she was forced to refer Kim and believes that she should have referred Kim from the beginning rather than taking her as a client.

REFERRAL THAT OCCURS DURING THE COUNSELING RELATIONSHIP

When There Is Countertransference

There are many reasons to consider referral after the therapeutic relationship begins. The most widely acknowledged reason to refer after the counseling relationship begins is countertransference. Countertransference occurs when the counselor assigns to the client attitudes and characteristics that do not belong to the client but rather belong (or belonged) to one of the counselor's significant others. More broadly, countertransference can also occur when a client hooks the counselor's own therapeutic issues. In either case, countertransference renders the counselor-client relationship nontherapeutic and therefore the counselor needs to refer the client to another therapist.

Counselors can feel that as long as they are in counseling themselves to deal with their countertransference issues, they do not have to refer their clients with whom they have countertransference. This judgment call depends upon the degree of countertransference, the types of issues, and the impact of the countertransference on the counseling relationship. Counselors who are well aware of their issues and who recognize when their countertransference issues become nontherapeutic are in a position to decide realistically when referral is necessary. Counselors who are not in touch with themselves and who believe that they have no countertransference issues are more likely to keep clients who should be referred and are more likely to blame the client when there is a lack of progress in therapy.

Supervision is the most valuable tool to keep an eye on countertransference. The supervisor can pick up issues to which the counselor is oblivious and also provides a sounding board for whether the client should be referred.

When There Is a Lack of Match

Another reason for referral after the counseling relationship has begun is the lack of personality match between the counselor and client. Each person has unique personality traits and some personalities do not match well enough to be therapeutic for the client. This does not mean that the counselor has countertransference issues or pathology that needs professional help. There is, in therapy, a "goodness of fit" where the right helper is matched with the right type of helpee. Cavanaugh (1980) likens the match to a suit of clothes. He asserts that there may be a beautiful suit of clothes at the store but it may be the wrong size, the wrong color, or a poor style for the particular figure type. He further asserts that when counselors are working on a professional level they should be selective about who they see. Counselors need to know themselves well enough to know with whom they are and are not effective.

Counselors, pastors, and other mental health professionals often have the erroneous belief that if they are mentally healthy, then they should be able to work with anyone. In the medical profession, a surgeon can operate on any person, no matter what the patient's personality, no matter whether the patient is motivated toward health or not, because the patient is anesthetized. However, in the helping professions, the personality match, the motivation, and the presenting problem all have a great bearing on the success of the counseling. Therefore, counselors need to be secure enough in themselves to be able to say when there is not a good fit. The counselor needs to believe that a lack of a good fit is neither the counselor's nor the client's fault but simply means that there is no therapeutic match. Then the counselor can be more therapeutic by referring the client to a therapist with whom he has more of an opportunity to find compatibility. If a counselor takes on clients who do not fit well with her style, then the counselor keeps on failing and the clients do too (Cavanaugh 1980).

Mental health professionals need to learn to let go of the misconception that they can help everyone. Even great baseball batters who hit .400 are failing to achieve first base six out of ten times at bat.

When Counseling Reaches an Impasse

Another reason for referral after a counseling relationship has begun is when the counselor and client feel that they are at an impasse. Through the therapeutic relationship, the counselor and client may have made great progress and then become stuck even though counselor and client both know that more growth is possible. Because counselors are human, housed in their own bodies, limited to their own perceptions and training, they can only take clients so far before a new perspective is needed. Supervision can often help when a counselor feels stumped and the client needs referral to another therapist.

Case Study: Therapeutic Impasse

> Larry is a pastoral counselor who had been seeing Gretchen for two years. When Gretchen first started seeing Larry, she was depressed, unemployed, and unhappy in her marriage, and had thought of suicide. Over the course of therapy, Larry and Gretchen worked on many of her issues. After two years, Gretchen was no longer suicidal, no longer suffered with depression, and was able to secure employment and work on her marriage with her husband. However, Gretchen knew that she still had some issues to address resulting from severe physical abuse as a child. Larry was feeling stuck. They had talked often about the abuse, but they seemed unable to move ahead. Gretchen and Larry agreed that they needed something different. Larry felt that he had failed Gretchen so he brought his concern to his supervisor. Through the supervisory session, Larry was able to affirm the work that he had done with Gretchen over the last two years and recognize that Gretchen needed a female counselor who was skilled in dealing with survivors of abuse in order to enhance the transference issues from Mom, the abuser, to the therapist. Larry was able to assist Gretchen in seeing her growth and in seeing that she deserved to address her final therapeutic issues with another therapist.

When the Counselor Discovers She Lacks Therapeutic Skills

A counselor also refers a client during counseling because she feels that she lacks the necessary therapeutic skills to aid the client's growth. Obviously, new counselors are frequently assessing their skill level to ascertain whether they can handle their clients' presenting and on-going problems. More experienced counselors also have limits to their skills. The field of counseling is so diverse, with specialization becoming more and more the means to expertise, that even experienced counselors may find themselves needing to refer to another who possesses skills in specialized areas. For example, career counselors refer mental health issues to mental health counselors; mental health counselors refer vocational rehabilitation issues to rehabilitation counselors.

Counselors who consider themselves generalists are often in the most difficult position to determine when their skill level is insufficient to help a client, because they have dedicated themselves to serving a variety of clients and presenting problems. Counselors can explore several feelings that may indicate that they are reaching the limits of their skills:

1. The counselor feels at a loss as to what techniques would help;
2. The counselor feels ineffective in her approach;
3. The client is not responding to the counselor's help;
4. The counselor cannot seem to understand the client's problem;
5. The counselor finds herself trying to read up on the client's issues to stay one step ahead of the client.

While the above symptoms may not predict a lack of skill level, they do identify feelings that counselors report when they feel that they are not on top of their counseling relationship with their client. Counselors who recognize their growing edges and feel empowered to refer are being therapeutic to their clients and are being honest with themselves.

When the Counselor is Sexually Attracted to the Client

The most perilous feeling that a counselor can have for a client is that of being sexually aroused by a client. Whether the client is being seductive or not, the counselor is held responsible by all helping professions' ethical codes to resist engaging in any seductive or sexual activity. A counselor who is sexually attracted to a client is approaching an area of temptation that can lead to litigation. In fact, one of the most frequent reasons for malpractice suits involving counselors is inappropriate sexual activity. The prudent counselor will refer any client for whom she feels sexual attraction.

REFERRAL THAT OCCURS UPON TERMINATION OF THE COUNSELING RELATIONSHIP

When the client and counselor agree on ending their therapeutic relationship, the client can fear being on his own without the counselor. There are options for termination that may soften the feeling of being turned loose with no support. For instance, referral to a group can provide support from peers and access to a therapist without the intensity of individual counseling, or if a client is ending his relationship with a therapist but for whatever reason would be unable to return to his original therapist if he should need additional counseling, then his therapist can give the client the name of another counselor for safety netting.

Case Study: Referral at Termination

> Jan had been in counseling with Denise for a year and felt very positive about the progress she made during that year. When Denise and Jan discussed termination, Jan felt ready to let go of her counseling relationship but felt that she would like to know that she could return if she needed to have more

counseling. Denise, however, was relocating to another city and would not be available to Jan if she should need further counseling. Denise provided Jan with an appropriate referral in case she should feel the need for further counseling. Jan felt more secure at termination knowing that she had the name of a competent counselor whom Denise respected.

When the Client Needs Help From Another Therapist

There are times when termination is occurring but the client feels that he still needs counseling. When a counselor feels that he has taken the client as far as she is willing, then the counselor will terminate the client while referring him for more counseling to another therapist. This occurs frequently when counselors specialize in crisis counseling. After working with the client in crisis, the client may need more counseling so the crisis counselor refers the client to a therapist who deals with longer term issues. A client who has been in crisis may need to change therapists before beginning longer term counseling, because once the crisis is over, the therapist who once helped the client through the crisis may be a constant reminder of the crisis and this reminder may interfere with the client's ability to move on to other issues. The client may be very grateful to the crisis counselor but still need a fresh start with a new counselor to address the longer term issues.

Hospitalization

Hospitalizing a client is a difficult decision and must be made in consultation with psychiatric medical personnel. The process of hospitalization is a subject for another book; the aspect of hospitalization relevant here is the fact that it must be viewed as a referral. Once the decision has been made to hospitalize a client, a psychiatrist will arrange for an inpatient bed at a hospital. The counselor or therapist at this point must let go of her client and let the hospital staff plan and execute the therapeutic plan that is applicable. Some hospitals encourage the counselor to maintain contact with the patient so that continuity is assured after hospitalization. If contact is maintained, the counselor has to recognize that the hospital staff is in charge of the patient's therapy while the patient is hospitalized. Because inpatient treatment is so different from outpatient, counselors tend to be very critical of hospital treatment, procedure, and medication. However, counselors who support the hospital and view the hospitalization as referral will be better able to work within the inpatient milieu.

Visitation by the counselor is often permitted and encouraged. However, this procedure can muddy the waters between the hospital's therapy and outpatient therapy. Therefore, the counselor has several choices: (1) not to visit the client, explaining to him that the hospital is now his therapeutic helper; (2) to visit the client but only talk about subjects that would be considered social; (3) to network with the hospital so that the counselor becomes a part of the therapeutic team and continues seeing the client in the hospital. Since the hospitalization is a referral, it is the hospital's responsibility to determine what role the counselor will play once the client becomes a patient.

After inpatient treatment, some hospitals refer to their own outpatient counselors while others will refer back to the original counselor for the patient's outpatient treatment. The hospital staff will decide whom their patient will see, with some input from the patient. The therapist needs to honor the hospital's choice of outpatient therapist, keeping the profile of a referring therapist and respecting the hospital as the therapeutic entity. In conclusion, the referral to a psychiatric hospital must be viewed by the therapist as any other referral: The therapist refers and then leaves the work to the referral source.

REFERRAL FOR NEUROPSYCHOLOGICAL EVALUATION

Mental health professionals need to be aware of instances in which clients should be referred for a neuropsychological evaluation. practitioners who are qualified to perform this type of evaluation are either psychiatrists or psychologists who have been specially trained in this field. Although the training and credentialling have not been well established, the American Psychological Association recognizes Division 40 as an interest group in this field. Counselors and other mental health professionals can also consult the International Neuropsychology Society and the National Academy of Neuropsychologist. While the American Board of Clinical Neuropsychology is the appropriate credentialling organization, there are so few in possession of the diplomate that it is elite and may exclude well-qualified persons (Lewis and Swiercinski, 1981). Therefore, finding a qualified person to do a neuropsychological evaluation requires the referring person to network with other mental health professionals in order to locate an appropriate professional to which a referral can be made.

Assessing Whether or Not Referral Is Necessary

Mental health professionals should watch for the signs and symptoms of possible neuropsychological problems. Ignoring this vital area can cause counselors to spend unnecessary time and energy treating a client who is not psychologically available to participate fully in the therapeutic process. Referral may be necessary if the counselor notes:

1. Aspects of the patient's developmental or medical history that suggest brain dysfunction;
2. The patient is complaining of symptoms that may indicate brain dysfunction;
3. That a cerebral disorder exists but questions whether there is a relevant impact on the patient's life and ability to function;
4. A client's seeming inability to facilitate treatment;
5. A client's need for rehabilitation counseling (the findings of a neuropsychological evaluation can be used to plan and monitor the effectiveness of cognitive retraining or any other therapeutic intervention);
6. Abrupt or progressive alterations in sensory, motor, emo-

tional, and cognitive functions that are not congruent with client's psychological diagnosis;

7. Longstanding or congenital dysfunction such as attention deficit disorders or learning disability;
8. A client's report of a head injury or stroke.

(Gouvier, Webster and Blanton, 1986; Horton and Sautter, 1986; Lewis, 1986; Rosenthal and Geckler, 1986; Lewis and Sinnett, 1987)

When making a referral for a neuropsychological evaluation, the same procedure can be followed as for any other referral. However, the counselor should take extra time and care to discuss thoroughly the reason for the referral and what to expect of the assessment, especially emphasizing that the process is not a physical or laboratory procedure. Further, the counselor should assure the client that the referral is for assessment and recommendation and that the client will return to the counselor to discuss the outcome of the assessment and the implementation of the recommendation.

The referring mental health professional should state the reasons for the referral and potential uses of the results to the neuropsychological evaluator. Communication should allow the evaluator to know whether the referral is for vocational planning, for academic potential, to determine the client's optimal treatment plan or to determine whether the client is able to benefit from outpatient counseling. The neuropsychologist would also benefit from information about the client's attitude toward the evaluation, the client's use of medications, and any other diagnostic evaluations that may have been performed.

4

The Client's Affective State During Referral

The referral process necessarily involves a myriad of feelings which can be helpful or deleterious to those involved in the referral. In some cases the affect may be overt, allowing for timely and open processing. But in other cases where affect may be covert, it is necessary to identify the feelings, accept the client's affect, process the feelings, and come to closure. Each client who is being referred has his own feelings about the process, depending on whether he instigated the referral, participated in the referral with his counselor, or is being referred over his opposition. The emotions listed below are discussed separately but in reality are multiply intertwined, so that the counselor must sort through various emotions to determine what is going on.

REJECTION

Clients enter counseling seeking an honest relationship where they can get an objective set of eyes on their problems in order to bring about positive change. The client's expectation that the relationship will develop into a caring bonding is necessary to the success of the counseling. However, this expectation sets the client up for rejection should the relationship not develop as expected. For many clients, their therapeutic relationship is the first honest, nonjudgmental relationship they have ever experienced. If, for whatever reason, the relationship should fail to develop, the client is vulnerable to experiencing the same rejected feeling which he may have experienced previously. The resultant reactions can be disappointment, depression, regression, blaming and anger. Because of the intensity of the reactions, many counselors hesitate to refer when one of their client's issues is continual rejection, even if the client does need a different therapist.

Rejection is a debilitating emotion and every person feels rejected at some time in her personal developmental career. However, the actual rejection is not the only activity that contributes to feelings of unworthiness and neglect. The feeling of rejection is exacerbated by negative self-talk, by lack of other support systems, and by lack of understanding surrounding the rejection.

A client who has experienced continual rejection during his life will experience referral as another form of rejection. The feeling cannot be removed but it can be openly discussed, understood, and accepted. If this occurs, the client's feeling may lose some of its sting and thus, he may begin the important process of emotional reframing of negative affect.

When a client feels rejected because of impending referral, the counselor need not rescind the referral. Instead, the referring counselor has the power to turn the referral into a therapeutic learning experience by:

1. Acknowledging the client's feeling of rejection as acceptable, realistic, and appropriate;
2. Reinforcing that appropriate referral is not rejection but is actually affirming of the client's self-worth;
3. Affirming that the client is an important person who deserves the best possible therapist for his problem;
4. Presenting the referral resource as one who is accepting of the client;

5. Reframing the referral as not a *personal* rejection but a *professional* decision;
6. Briefly exploring the pattern of rejection in the client's life history, outlining why the client looks for and assumes rejection in relationships.

BETRAYAL

Betrayal is a kindred emotion to rejection. Like rejection, the feeling of betrayal communicates unworthiness or disappointment to the client. A client who feels betrayed by his counselor also may feel rejected through the betrayal. Unlike rejection, betrayal is usually expressed outwardly toward the counselor ("You did this to me") rather than being directed inwardly (I have been rejected). Betrayal surfaces during referral when the client feels that his counselor has built a pseudo-relationship while the client has entrusted his entire psychological health to the counselor. In other words, the client feels that the counselor is not as invested in the counseling relationship as the client. Why else would the counselor be willing to refer him? Betrayal can be built on a dependency need and taps Erikson's earliest stage of Trust versus Mistrust. Clients who react to referral by feeling betrayed are clients who have trouble with intimate relationships because they consistently term any motivation of another as betrayal. They express their feeling of betrayal as self-righteous anger and with an attitude of naturally expecting this type of behavior because everyone else has betrayed their infantile trust.

The statement that is usually expressed when betrayal is the issue is, "I counted on you to help me and you are not doing as you promised; therefore, you have betrayed the trust and hope that I placed in you." When the client expresses betrayal, the counselor may feel the need to defend herself, which in turn signifies to the client that his assumption of betrayal is accurate. When a client feels betrayed during the referral process, the counselor need not defend her behavior. Instead, the counselor can facilitate the therapeutic referral process by:

1. Listening attentively to the feelings being expressed by the client;
2. Accepting the fact that the client feels betrayed;
3. Allowing the client catharsis, if anger is present;
4. Helping the client identify another time in his life when he felt betrayed (how is this feeling the same as or different from the past feeling?);
5. Identifying exactly what behaviors or conditions existed that triggered the feeling of betrayal and discussing openly, without defensiveness, how the behaviors or conditions may be something other than betrayal.

Thus, the referring counselor can utilize the client's negative feeling of betrayal to effect a change in attitude, making the referral process a therapeutic endeavor.

There is one caution regarding betrayal which the counselor needs to keep in mind. If a client is being referred and the counselor shares client information with the referral resource prematurely or shares information that the client feels is unnecessary for the referral process, then the client may justifiably feel betrayed. When to share information and how much information to share when making a referral is covered in other chapters of this book.

DISAPPOINTMENT

Clients entering counseling are placing their trust in a stranger. The relationship that ensues can cause the client to place the counselor on a pedestal of respect and admiration. Sometimes the pedestal can be constructed before the counselor and client even meet, if the referral source has built the counselor's reputation up to the client. If the counselor then needs to refer the client, the client can feel a sense of loss: loss of hope, loss of confidence, loss of a potential relationship, disappointment.

Clients most likely to respond to referral in this way are clients who have invested a great deal of hope in this new counseling relationship because previous counseling relationships have not proven helpful. The client's primary response is "I didn't really think this would work. I wonder if there is anyone who can help me." He is skeptical about the new referral but willing to listen to the counselor's opinion. The danger of this stated response is that it may prompt the counselor to assure the client that there is indeed help for him and that this new referral will be the one. The client then leaves the counselor hopeful for the new relationship, already setting the new counselor up on a pedestal, and setting himself up for more disappointment should the situation not work out this time either. Clients who present themselves in this repetitive cycle of hope, disappointment, and hope again are clients who are dependent.

Counselors can assist clients who express the emotion of disappointment by:

1. Letting the client express his feelings of disappointment;
2. Identifying the loss of confidence as grief work;
3. Assisting the client to see the counselor as human, with limitations and assets that do not match his needs;
4. Pointing out the self-defeating repetitive cycle of hopefulness, disappointment, hopefulness, disappointment, etc.;
5. Not assuring the client that the new counselor is the perfect match;
6. Assisting the client in not putting the new counselor on a pedestal by identifying the referral counselor's realistic strengths and growing edges.

Clients are then in a better position to enter the new therapeutic relationship.

FEAR

Clients who express fear upon the first mention of referral do so because a referral changes an intimate relationship. Fear is a difficult emotion to deal with therapeutically because fear can immobilize a client, thus rendering the referral moot. Some clients will openly express their fear and are eager to address their concerns. However, others will terminate with their counselor and accept the referral information with no intention of following through even though they promise their counselor that they will make the contact. Such a client quickly accepts the referral with no questions asked. He appears to be the ideal referred client because he accepts the referral, readily agrees with the counselor's assessment, and looks eager to get started, but then he never follows through. Clients acting in such a manner need to be carefully assessed. They will often not receive the counseling that they need out of fear. In fact, until their immobilizing fear is worked through, they should not be referred. This type of client is often better off with his original counselor, whom he has grown to trust and with whom he feels a sense of comfort, than with no counselor at all. However, if the client needs a different counselor, then his current counselor must spend some extra time to address the client's fear before the referral is attempted. Some suggestions for dealing with this situation:

1. The ease with which the client accepts the referral should not deter the counselor from exploring feelings of fear.
2. The counselor may have to suggest the label of "fear" to the client as an emotion that is perfectly normal and acceptable.
3. The counselor can suggest that the client visualize how he felt when he first received the suggestion of counseling with her. There should have been some of the same feeling of fear, but the client obviously overcame the fear and made the contact and then followed through. Since the client has had at least one success in overcoming his fear and this time it paid off, then the client has proven his ability to manage fear. The counselor can build on the first success in getting the client to reduce his fear and encourage him to risk again.
4. The counselor can utilize systematic dissertation to reduce the anxiety which usually accompanies fear.
5. The new therapist can be brought into a session with the referring counselor and client so that the client can meet his new counselor in a safe atmosphere.

Clients who express fear of referral due to the belief that they are unlovable and may never find Mr. or Ms. Right Counselor need to look at their fear as self-defeating and catastrophizing. While the suggestions will help with the referral, the referring counselor also needs to identify the fear of never finding the right therapist as a therapeutic issue. This enables the client to look at his fear as something to be worked through not just for this referral, but for his lifetime. Connecting his fear of referral to his other fears of failure will help the client see that this fear is just one of the symptoms of larger issues which he needs to work on to achieve a more positive mental health. This tactic may not actually reduce the fear as the above suggestions do, but it may motivate the client to act on the referral despite his fear, in order to acquire better mental health.

ANXIETY

While fear is usually an overpowering emotion that can immobilize a client, anxiety is often a less debilitating emotion that is more apt to be present in all client. Clients express anxiety verbally by asking questions that entail who, what, when, where, and how much answers. At first glance, the client may appear to be looking for an excuse for not accepting the referral. In some instances, this may indeed be the case. However, usually clients are simply trying to collect as much information as possible in order to quiet their anxiety.

Despite the nebulous nature of anxiety, this emotion can cause clients to excuse themselves from acting or, at least, can cause clients to postpone their action. Therefore, anxiety needs to be dealt with during the referral process if the referral process is to be a therapeutic learning experience.

1. Counselors can utilize many of the fear-reduction techniques that were listed above. Of particular use is systematic desensitization and anxiety-fear reduction roleplay.

2. When clients feel anxious, they need as much information as possible. Therefore, allowing the clients to ask as many questions about the referral and the referral resources as possible will often assist in anxiety reduction.

3. Anxiety also responds well to guided imagery and mental rehearsal.

4. Anxiety is a part of everyday life and change. Helping the client to accept anxiety as totally natural will allow the client to think of himself as "normal" and may assist him in not allowing the referral anxiety to monopolize his life.

ANGER

Clients who express anger at being referred are often covering up other emotions. Anger is usually an emotion that allows the client to express safer emotions outwardly while masking truer feelings which would be too painful to experience. It is, therefore, important to help the client to translate the anger into the deeper emotions. This process is very therapeutic for the client and can assist him in his next counseling experience, if he has used his referral to uncover his truer emotions. Anger can mask rejection, betrayal, lack of self-worth, worry, depression, fear, and anxiety. For example, if a client says "Why are you referring me? I thought we were finally getting somewhere," the counselor can translate this into "Why are you rejecting me? I think we worked well together. I trust you." While the exact wording may vary with each client and his specific presenting problem, the counselor needs to look for the deeper meaning behind the anger and assist the client in expressing his true feelings about the referral.

Some examples of angry statements by clients that have been successfully translated into the deeper feelings are presented below. Each statement or question by the client was stated in an extremely angry manner, but expletives have been deleted.

Case One

CLIENT (anger): I feel bounced around by you guys.

COUNSELOR (going deeper): It must feel as if no one wants to work with you.

CLIENT (worry and fear): Yea. Do you see me as a troubled person?

COUNSELOR: I see you as a person with troubles. And these troubles need a special kind of help.

CLIENT (grief): I guess you're the first person who has really listened to me and I don't want to lose that.

COUNSELOR: I understand, but you deserve the best help possible and I am not that person.

CLIENT: OK, I trust you. But if this doesn't work out with Stan [the referral resource], can I come back to you?

COUNSELOR: If you and Stan really work hard at your relationship and it doesn't work, then I'd like to hear from you so that I can make another appropriate referral for you. OK?

CLIENT: OK.

Case Two

CLIENT (anger): You are trying to get rid of me!

COUNSELOR: (going deeper); You feel I'm rejecting you?

CLIENT (anger, yielding to rejection): You *are* rejecting me! What are you trying to do, get rid of some of your worst cases?

COUNSELOR: Are you afraid that you are one of my worst cases?

CLIENT: I've always been the worst at everything. I was always chosen last in gym class. I was always the last kid my parents thought of, and now you are doing the same thing.

COUNSELOR: Actually, I'm affirming you.

CLIENT (questioning): Huh?

COUNSELOR: I am referring you to the *best* alcohol rehabilitation clinic in this area because I want you to have the opportunity to get well.

CLIENT: I didn't think of it that way.

Case Three

CLIENT (anger mixed with teasing): How dare you take this promotion, leaving me to someone less experienced.

COUNSELOR (going deeper): Do you feel I'm rejecting you because of my promotion?

CLIENT (crying and grieving): Not necessarily rejecting me, but I feel that you didn't think about me when you took the job.

COUNSELOR: I took a long time to think about you and who you would work best with. I have arranged for you to see one of the most experienced people on our staff.

CLIENT (sensing betrayal): Oh, I bet I was the subject of a long discussion.

COUNSELOR: As a matter of fact, I only asked Jill [the referral resource] if she could take another client. I wanted to talk with you first.

CLIENT (intrigued and hope returning): What's Jill like?

In each of the above scenarios, the client began angry and through affirmation, careful questioning, and deeper exploration of feelings began to explore his or her emotions underneath the anger. Also in each case, some resolution to the referral begins but more grieving and disengagement is still needed. Referral and its accompanying feelings and grief take time and processing if the referral is to be therapeutic.

When the client presents anger at being referred, the counselor can assist the client by:

1. Listening to and accepting the anger;
2. Not becoming defensive;
3. Asking a question about a deeper feeling that may be covered up by the anger;
4. Affirming the client's right to his feeling;
5. Standing firm on the referral while still being available to the client in the present to work on his concerns about the referral.

DEPRESSION

Although depression is a part of the grieving process which usually accompanies referral, depression can also be exhibited as a sole reaction to the prospect of being referred. This particularly happens when the client has experienced depression previously and is now hopeful or is feeling better at the time of referral. Counselors who must refer clients who are working on depression need to expect a recurrence of depression as a reaction to the referral. Depression is the mode of reaction to change of these clients, and referral will be no exception. Because depressive episodes can trigger suicidal ideation, referral of depressed clients must be very carefully handled. Depressed clients who are making progress with their current therapist should be referred only if absolutely necessary. The counseling relationship is so critical to these clients that referral can send them spiraling into a major depressive episode with suicidal ideation.

However, if referral is necessary, then the interruption of the hopeless-helpless cycle that is so indicative of depression is critical. The hopeless portion of the cycle is usually expressed with such statements as:

"No one can ever help me."
"My problems are too overwhelming."
"I feel totally empty inside."
"What's the use?"
"I should just give up."

In response to the hopeless side of the cycle, the referring counselor must help the client to see hope in the referral where currently the client sees none. The following helps clients with their hopelessness:

1. If progress has been made in the current counseling relationship, then this progress becomes the symbol of hope that counseling is working. If progress was made once, it can be made again.
2. Focus on the client's hard work in counseling as that which

made the difference. Clients are in the counseling session typically one hour per week and are away from counseling 167 hours per week. What clients do with their time outside of counseling is extremely important.

3. Identify the hopeless feeling as a part of the depression and not a result of the client's life-style or the referral.

4. Use cognitive techniques such as thought stopping or thought substitution to assist the client in thinking differently about the referral.

The helpless portion of the depressive cycle is usually expressed with statements such as:

"I can't do this alone."
"I try, but I don't seem to get anywhere."
"When I try, someone else always destroys my progress."

In response to the helpless side of the cycle, the referring counselor must help the client to see the help that can be his. The following assists clients with their helplessness:

1. Point out that the client is not helpless. He has sought help through counseling and that action empowers him.

2. Focus on whatever else the client has accomplished on his own outside the counseling relationship, for example, a decision he made or an activity in which he has participated.

3. Use cognitive restructuring techniques to substitute empowering thoughts for disabling thoughts.

Depression is a very serious response to life stressors. In referral, depression can trigger suicide and manipulation to stop the referral process. Counselors need to weigh carefully the risk of the client's reaction when considering referral. Referral of a depressed client is more appropriate at the beginning or ending of a counseling relationship where the relationship either has not formed or is naturally coming to closure. A depressed client has usually suffered a great deal of rejection and betrayal but has chosen to turn the feelings on himself. If he is able to form a therapeutic relationship, then that becomes that most important relationship in his life. To refer such a client may cause severe consequences; therefore, a great deal of care must be exercised.

RELIEF

When a client feels that he is not developing a therapeutic relationship with the therapist, then his response to being referred may be relief. The client will appreciate the referral more than the counseling. Perhaps the strongest emotional reaction will be the counselor's feeling of failure, which is discussed in other chapters of this book.

Clients who feel relieved at having been referred receive the news of referral with interest. They seem anxious to get started and ask appropriate questions. In fact, they often respond to referral in much the same manner as clients who are afraid and have no intention of following through. The major difference between the two reactions is usually in the affective way they ask questions. Clients who are afraid of referral receive the information and ask appropriate questions, agreeing to follow through, but usually their affect is somewhat blunted or aloof. Clients who are relieved and interested in the possibility of referral appear open, interactive, and willing to communicate.

Relief can also be experienced by the family of the client when the referral involves much-needed hospitalization or admittance to a specialized inpatient clinic. The client, however, may not be feeling relieved at all. Instead, the client may be experiencing any one of the other feelings mentioned in this chapter. Therefore, the counselor may have to respond differently to the client than to his family.

When the client expresses relief, the counselor may have some difficulty in dealing with him because of her own feelings of failure. Listen to the client and affirm his feeling that the relationship is not working or that another specialist is needed. If the counselor is able to avoid feeling personally responsible for the lack of a therapeutically "good fit" in the relationship, then the client can feel relief because his therapist is not being hurt by the referral.

A client often knows when a relationship is not therapeutic and dreads having to bring this to his therapist's attention. He will then either drift away, making excuses as to why he cannot continue in counseling (usually he will talk about money or time) or he confronts his fears and openly brings the problem to the therapist. The feeling of relief can come either because he has confronted the issue and is relieved that it is out in the open or because his therapist accepts his feelings without defensiveness.

ANTICIPATION

Another feeling that clients have during the referral process is one of anticipation. Anticipation can have many of the qualities of anxiety, but without a negative connotation. There is a sense of hope about anticipation that is absent in anxiety. A counselor should look for this feeling as a sign that the referral process has acquired a positive valence to the client. As clients work through their negative feelings of rejection, betrayal, anger, etc., they begin to anticipate working with a new counselor. They will often question their current counselor about their new therapist or therapeutic setting. The referring counselor can take pleasure in answering the client's questions and know that the time has come for the actual transfer to take place.

GRIEF

Grieving over the loss of the therapeutic relationship is a part of all referrals where the relationship has been established and has facilitated client growth. Elizabeth Kübler-Ross has written extensively on the grieving process in death and dying. The five stages of grief that Ross has delineated also can take place during referral.

Working through the grieving process takes time and often the referral must be accomplished long before the entire grieving process has been completed. Therefore, the counselor needs to accept the client at whatever stage he is in at the time and encourage him to explore his feelings at all five stages. Some of the affective expressions of referral at each stage are slightly different from those of death and dying. For example, instead of expressing "I cannot believe this is happening to me" in the denial stage of death and dying, a client may say "I cannot believe that I will not be seeing you every week." In the bargaining stage, instead of "God, if you let me live until my grandchild is born, I'll give all my money to the church," a client might say "If I take the referral, can I be in one of your groups?" Acceptance will probably look more like anticipation than the giving up or peace of dying. Anger and depression have been covered earlier in this chapter. All in all, grieving cannot be rushed, but should be expressed and accepted as a part of referral.

NO REACTION

When a client seems to have no reaction to the news of referral, there are two possible reasons: He was not invested in the relationship, or he has shut down his feelings successfully in order to escape them.

If the client was not invested in the therapy, then referral is appropriate and may even be welcomed and expected. This is particularly true when the relationship is in the early stages and is not working. Usually both client and counselor are aware of the problem and the feeling is mutual. In some cases, the counselor may be deluded in thinking that there is a relationship when in fact the counselor is the only one working at the alliance. In this scenario, the counselor will be quite surprised at the client's lack of reaction to the referral. The therapist then wonders what it was that she did wrong, that the relationship did not develop. However, a counselor cannot expect to work well with every client, even though she desires it. The client's lack of reaction may be a key to the lack of this relationship. Supervision also helps counselors to have a third set of eyes on the therapeutic progress and can aid counselors in working through their feelings about referral.

The second reason for the lack of a reaction to referral is that the client's affective state may be shut down or denied. This problem will take many sessions to work through and would be beyond the scope of the referral process. However, if the referral is to be therapeutic, then the counselor can attempt to lay some groundwork for the next therapist by:

1. Asking the client what he is *feeling* about the referral (if he says "Nothing," then ask what he *thinks* about the referral).
2. Pointing out that clients have a variety of reactions to being referred and exploring the various feelings and thoughts that are frequently reported;
3. Explaining that these feelings are "normal," appropriate, and healthy;
4. Modeling the activity of feeling by expressing an honest emotion about having to refer the client (for example, "I feel sad that we will not have the opportunity to work together").

The above may begin the spadework necessary to allow the client the freedom to own his feelings. The rest of the work will be accomplished with the new referral resource.

POSITIVE FEELINGS ABOUT REFERRAL

There are times when referral is necessary and accepted by the client. The client is grateful and pleased with the counselor's interaction and their relationship. At this point, clients are often verbal about their gratitude and will compliment the counselor on the work she has done. Counselors should accept these feelings of gratitude without embarrassment and without discounting the client's feelings. Clients need to have their positive as well as negative feelings affirmed. When a client is exuding his enthusiasm and respect for the counselor, it can be difficult to receive the feelings. The counselor should:

1. Openly appreciate the compliments;
2. Affirm that both client and counselor worked hard;
3. Say thank you;
4. Refrain from telling the client that the counselor is just a catalyst and that the client did all the work (this discounts the valuable part that the counselor played and denigrates the positive therapeutic relationship);
5. Show the client where the power of the therapy lies and why counseling works so he can appreciate himself, the counselor, and the therapeutic alliance.

CONCLUSION

Clients' feelings toward being referred are varied and often complicated. One client can express all the various emotions discussed in this chapter during the referral process. Counselors need to see referral as a part of therapy and utilize the referral in such a way that the client can learn and grow not only from the experience of referral but also from his own feelings and reactions. In this way, the referral process is not just transferring a client from one clinician to another or deferring to one who has more experience but instead is a continuation of the therapeutic process of growth.

5

The Counselor's Affective State During Referral

Counselors are not immune to emotions when involved with making a referral. Although the counselor will tend to concentrate on the client's affective state, she needs to recognize, acknowledge, and work through her own feelings involving the referral of a client, when that referral is the result of difficulty with the counseling relationship. When the therapist's emotions are evident, she can seek to work through the feelings with her supervisor, with a colleague, in a staff meeting, or in her own therapy.

Perhaps this is the place to affirm the absolute necessity for all helpers to be connected in some way to other helpers, either through supervision, collegial sharing, consultation, or personal counseling. Just as clients need another set of eyes on their problems, so do counselors need an objective viewpoint on their interactions with their clients. Obviously, the newer the counselor is to the field,d the more intense and formalized the supervision and the consultation needs to be. However, helpers never outgrow the need for supervision/consultation.

The referral of a clients can evoke feelings of failure, guilt, anger, fear, rejection, and grief and open the door to questioning one's own competence. These feelings are difficult to own and it is tempting to ignore them because of the painful questions that must be asked. However, if counselors expect their clients to own, understand, and work through emotions, can the counselors expect less of themselves?

Clients expect their counselors to be healthier than themselves. While this may or may not be an erroneous assumption, the expectation certainly is that counselors should be aware of their own personal therapeutic issues and willing to face their own pathology and needs. The need to refer taps the counselor's issues and often exacerbates the need for supervision or consultation.

FAILURE

The word *failure* implies that the counselor was lacking, inadequate, or insufficient in the counseling relationship and therefore disappointed those who were depending on her. The most frequent feeling that counselors express when they find that they need to refer a client is failure. There are many reasons to refer a client that do not evoke failure, such as the practice being at the maximum capacity, the therapist moving or changing jobs, or the client being in need of a different type of counseling that is outside the counselor's ken. However, counselors who struggle with a client, work hard, and see little progress tend to place blame for the failure of the relationship on themselves and see themselves as inadequate or unsuccessful.

There can be many reasons for the counseling relationship to fail, to develop, or thrive:

1. The counselor may have countertransference issues with the client.
2. The counselor may not have the particular skills needed to deal with the client at this time.

3. The counselor may be overinvested in other relationships that are demanding and exhausting.

4. The client and counselor may not be an appropriate therapeutic match, i.e.:
   a. The client may need a different theoretical style than the counselor's style.
   b. The client may not respond to the counselor's personality in a therapeutic manner.
   c. The counselor may not respond therapeutically to the client's personality.
   d. The counselor may not be interested in working with the client's presenting problem.

5. The client may either be sabotaging the relationship or not be motivated to invest in the relationship.

Countertransference

The counselor's feelings of failure when a therapeutic relationships fails to thrive are debilitating and often exaggerated. Perhaps the greatest feeling of failure comes when countertransference issues are present. Counselors like to feel that they are in control of themselves and the therapy. Countertransference occurs when the counselor assigns to a client thoughts, feelings, and attitudes that belong to one of the counselor's significant others, which signals to the counselor that she is not totally in control and that her personal issues are evident.

When countertransference occurs and referral is appropriate, the counselor needs to:

1. Acknowledge that all helpers have countertransference issues which, from time to time, interfere with their ability to be therapeutic;
2. Forgive herself for being a human being with emotions and painful experiences;
3. Identify exactly what the countertransference issues are, and

understand their etiology and triggering mechanisms and circumstances (this may require personal therapy).

4. Restate the feeling of failure in terms of ordinary and normal reactions that will occur from time to time to any therapist;

5. Express the problem with a sense of humor at her own humanity;

6. Note if her various countertransference issues seem to be emerging frequently and seek supervision and counseling if she ascertains that she has been experiencing difficulty with several therapeutic relationships. (This requires that the counselor know herself well and be able to assess her relationships and personal issues honestly. Counselors who are unable to do this honest assessment will find themselves having a roller-coaster effect in their therapeutic relationships.)

When considering whether a referral is in order because of countertransference issues, the counselor needs to examine several critical areas.

1. The counselor needs to identify the countertransference issue. Is the issue as simple as a resemblance between the client and someone the counselor knows and loves? Or does the client trigger negative angry reactions in the counselor because the client reacts to life exactly as the counselor's mother did?

2. Once the countertransference is identified, the counselor should assess the intensity of her reaction. Obviously, countertransference caused by a client who physically resembles a significant other in the counselor's life is not of the same intensity or danger to the relationship as countertransference that is fraught with negative affective valences.

3. The assessment of the intensity of the countertransference will then lead the counselor to consider whether referral is imperative. The rule of thumb is: If the countertransference interferes with the counselor's ability to be therapeutic with the client, then the client needs to be referred. Sometimes the countertransference may be intense but positive. Even though the countertransference is positive, however, it may still interfere with the counselor's ability to

be therapeutic. For example, if the counselor feels deep love for her brother, and the client looks and acts like her brother, then the therapist may be unable to confront him about his self-defeating behavior. The relationship may feel wonderful and still not be therapeutic.

Approaching the client about referral when the counselor is experiencing countertransference is difficult. On one hand, counselors feel that they owe the client the truth, but on the other hand they may want to prevent the client from seeing their own vulnerability. The most effective way to approach a client who has triggered countertransference is to tell the client that the therapeutic relationship has not developed as the counselor had hoped and that another counselor would be of benefit to the client. Further, the counselor should explain that the relationship is the most important contributor to successful therapy and the client deserves the best chance at developing that relationship. If the client asks for specific reasons why, the counselor should answer his questions generally but truthfully. With some clients, the counselor may need to go as far as saying that the client's presence is stirring up emotions in her that are demanding much time and energy to sort through and therefore the client is not receiving the most timely support he deserves. The counselor can point out that all clients evoke emotional responses in their counselors but sometimes, because of human nature, the reactions are stronger and more time-consuming. However, avoid talking about the concept as countertransference and its ramifications.

Lack of Skills

If the counselor does not have the particular skills needed to deal with the client, then the counselor may talk to herself in a negative manner in terms of "should," "ought," and "if only."

Newly trained counselors accept that they have acquired counseling skills but need supervised experience in order to gain the confidence they need. During those first few years after training, new counselors are overly sensitive to the fact that they lack experience and skills in dealing with every type of presenting problem and may quickly refer when they perceive that they are in over their heads with a client. However, there are times when a new counselor takes a client who has presenting problems with which she feels comfortable and then discovers, once the helping relationship is established, that the client's problems require a higher skill level. The novice counselor then sees herself as a failure and loses sight of the fact that referral has to occur because of her novice status rather than any failure of her own or of the counseling relationship. Positive self talk, continued education experience, and supervision will help the novice to assess her skills realistically and become more seasoned as a counselor.

Sometimes the newly trained counselor in such a situation may be advised by her supervisor that she should not refer the client but rather work with the client utilizing intensive supervision. Thus, the helping relationship is maintained and the client benefits from the relationship as well as the supervisor's expertise. In addition, the counselor gains skills in dealing with a difficult presenting problem. The client deserves the most excellent help possible, ethically counselors must see that clients are connected with the appropriate therapist. (See chapter on ethical concerns.) However, sometimes the most appropriate counselor is not the most trained but the one who has the trusting relationship with the client.

Another problem new counselors face is that of making a critical mistake that leads to referral. The temptation is for the counselor to blame herself for the error and tell herself that a more experienced counselor would not have made the error. A new counselor needs to look at each mistake as a learning experience and not assume that her inexperience caused the error. Mistakes are made by experienced counselors, too.

Case Study: Counselor Error Leads to Referral

Estelle made contact with Joyce, a counselor who had two years of postmaster's experience. Joyce was just beginning to

> feel some confidence in her skills. Estelle presented a problem which Joyce had handled before — anxiety disorder with occasional panic attacks. After four sessions, Estelle reported feeling less anxious. At the fifth session, Estelle did not show up, so after twenty minutes, Joyce called Estelle's home. Estelle was not home but her husband answered the phone. Joyce said, "Hello, this is Joyce (Last Name) from (Community) Counseling Services calling. Is Estelle home?" The husband said that she was not. Joyce said, "Estelle had an appointment with me at 4:00. Do you know if she left for the appointment?" Estelle's husband said that he did not know where Estelle was and then asked what type of counseling the agency provided. Joyce said "Individual counseling. I'll call Estelle later to reschedule." Joyce never had another session with Estelle. Later that day Estelle called and told Joyce that she had not told her husband that she was in counseling, that she felt betrayed, that she and her husband had had a donnybrook over the deception, and that she could not come back. Estelle did thank Joyce for her help in alleviating some of her anxiety and promptly terminated. Joyce was absolutely devastated. It had never occurred to her that Estelle had kept her counseling a secret from her husband and it had never occurred to her that telling a client's spouse that his wife was in counseling was a breech of confidentiality. Joyce was very hard on herself. She said that she had broken a client's confidence and should never be entitled to a client's trust again.

Many counselors, both novice and experienced, have made this mistake, though perhaps without the extreme result of the client terminating therapy. Through working with her supervisor, Joyce finally saw that she had helped Estelle, that she had fallen into a trap and made an error in judgment, and that if she learned from it, she could be a better, more experienced counselor. Joyce forgave herself and continued learning.

Experienced counselors are even more likely to flagellate themselves when they must refer due to lack of skills. Experienced counselors have gained confidence and skill in working with clients to whom they are well suited. However, occasionally an experienced counselor encounters a difficult client, one who either presents a problem the counselor knows she cannot handle or presents such a complex of multiple problems that the therapist feels overwhelmed. The experienced counselor who supervises novice counselors who revere her expertise, may find it especially difficult to acknowledge the limits of her own competency. When that counselor is then faced with referral due to lack of skills, the pedestal of exaggerated expectation which she herself may have begun to accept, begins to shake.

It is absurd to believe that experience means that one knows everything or, at least, can handle all presenting problems. The counselor who believes that she *should* be able to handle any type of situation is falling into a self-deceiving trap which can only lead to feelings of inadequacy. The counselor who knows her skills and limitations and refers easily based on her own self-knowledge and her colleagues' complementary skills, will avoid setting herself up for feelings of failure.

A counselor who can assess her skills and refer when a client's problems surpass her skills, creates an empowering and therapeutic milieu for herself and her client. However, even an experienced counselor can be trapped into believing that her skills are appropriate to the task only to discover that the presenting problem is not the real issue. Then, in the middle of building the counseling relationship, she is faced with the problem of referral. The counselor must then acknowledge not only her lack of necessary skills, but also her incorrect assessment of the client's initial presentation of the problem.

The counselor who can see these difficult times as a necessary part of a counselor's career process can take them in stride, and even expect to learn from them. Experienced counselors as well as novices can use supervision effectively when referring due to lack of skills in a certain area. Supervision can give the counselor support, assist the counselor in emotionally resolving the feelings of failure, and aid the counselor in deciding which referral resources to use. (See chapter on supervision.)

Referring Too Quickly

Although this book is about how to make referral therapeutic, in some cases referral may not be the most appropriate therapeutic choice for a client. The ability to know when not to refer is an essential aspect of any therapist's referral skills. Any novice or experienced counselor can refer clients who seem too difficult for them to handle. However, supervisor's need to watch for the counselor who gives up too quickly on a client, especially on specific types of clients. This can signal unresolved countertransference issues, misguided faith in the power of others, or lack of confidence in her own therapeutic skills. The counselor who refers prematurely may consider it easier to refer a client than to have to deal with countertransference issues or to learn new skills. (See chapter on supervision.)

Counselors Who Do Not Refer

A counselor may refuse to refer a client even though she is experiencing countertransference or not skilled enough to work with the client. Counselors who take this posture are overconfident; believing themselves capable of handling all clients, and they are unable to admit their shortcomings. Supervisors need to identify and intervene with this counselor's refusing to consider referral when the client would benefit from the referral. This reluctance to refer may reflect unresolved therapeutic issues requiring attention. There are ethical issues involved when a counselor retains clients despite the need to refer which will be discussed in other sections of this book. See Chapters 9 and 10 in this book.

Overextension

At times, any counselor can become overextended in her professional career and personal life. However, when a counselor refers a client or prospective client because she feels overwhelmed by the energy needed to attend to her own issues, the counselor may experience a feeling of failure. Counselors, psychologists, psychiatrists, and other helpers who assist others in managing their time and energy, may expect that they themselves will always manage their own time, energy, and relationships perfectly. When counselors find their own personal and professional energy depleted, they often feel that they are failing to manage their own lifestyles. If they then must refer clients, they feel they are failing their clients too.

Counselors who find themselves in this dilemma need to work through their challenge and emerge stronger counselors by:

1. Acknowledging that this stressful period is typical of all human beings, even helpers;
2. Calling on their skills and knowledge of human behavior and personal management to work through their personal and professional issues;
3. Prioritizing their needs and making knowledgeable, therapeutic referrals of new clients or current clients who would be better served by other therapists;
4. Making the commitment to take care of themselves so that they can in turn assist others to do the same;
5. Eliminating the word *failure* from their vocabulary and refusing to accept that they have failed.

An overextended counselor needs to see that her referral of prospective clients is therapeutic for the clients because they will be placed in the hands of a counselor who is available to build a helping relationship, and is therapeutic for the counselor because she will bring her energy and time commitment within her own grasp.

Lack of Therapeutic Match

Since each client and each counselor has a unique personality paradigm, the counselor embraces her own therapeutic style and the client has his own way of responding to therapy. There will be times when a counselor's theoretical approach will not match the client's need for a specific type of interactive style. A counselor who is faced with the decision to refer a client because he is not responding therapeutically to her style will often internalize the irreconcilable differences as her failure to positively interact and build a relationship with her client. However, this lack of therapeutic match is not the fault of either the client or the counselor; it is simply a fact. The therapeutic relationship is a form of marriage in which the personality match is important. In a marriage, each person brings unique talents to the relationship. Prior to the marriage, there is a period of engagement in which the couple tests their commitment to the relationship and decides whether they each feel that the relationship is healthy for them. So, too, in a therapeutic relationship there is a period of engagement and trust-building before the client enters the therapeutic middle phase. During the engagement phase, both client and counselor are deciding whether they can work together. When the answer is affirmative, then the therapeutic relationship receives commitment. If the answer is negative, neither the counselor nor the client has failed. However the counselor still has the responsibility of assessing the reason why the relationship did not develop and of assisting the client with a therapeutic referral to another counselor who may be capable of forming a therapeutic relationship with the client.

Case Study: Mismatched Client and Counselor

> John is a thirty-five-year-old psychiatrist who approaches his clients in a highly interactive, spontaneous, verbal manner. He uses insight therapy in which he frequently poses his interpretation. John is an extremely gregarious person who fills any void in a conversation with his own thoughts and feelings.
>
> Betsy is a twenty-nine-year-old woman who is studying to become a social worker. As a part of her course of study, Betsy decided to treat herself to therapy, knowing that she had a few issues to resolve. Betsy processes information very slowly. One of her graduate student colleagues commented that he could almost see her wheels turning as she thought. Betsy is insightful, pensive, and very quiet. She only speaks after she has thought through all of her response options and then consciously decided what her response would be.
>
> John and Betsy met for three sessions and both came away

> feeling totally frustrated with their relationship. John said that Betsy was so quiet and passive that he felt that he was doing all the work. He was bored, tired, and wanted to refer her. Betsy said that John was not giving her room to process. She said that he always filled the silence and she felt pressured, misunderstood, and frustrated. She wanted a referral.
>
> Obviously, this couple could not establish a therapeutic relationship without one of them making a serious personality alteration. They processed cognitive and emotional information differently. John felt as if he had failed at the relationship. He had prided himself on being able to bond quickly with any client. Betsy also felt badly that she had finally tried therapy and it had not worked. Betsy was referred to a counselor with client-centered style, and felt very comfortable with her new counselor. John used the incident to learn about himself and the type of client with whom he does not easily engage.

In the above example, neither counselor nor client responded in a therapeutic way to the other's personality. It is possible that the counselor may feel comfortable with the client but the client does not feel at ease with the counselor or vice versa. Whether the mismatch is one-sided or, as in the case study, both are feeling uncomfortable with the relationship, referral becomes necessary.

Finally, there may be a mismatch between counselor and client as to the interest in the presenting problem. As much as counselors pride themselves on being excellent listeners and compassionate helpers, a counselor may discover that she is not always interested in her client's problem. A counselor, however, may feign interest, telling herself that she should be interested because the client is in pain and she should look beyond the initial subject matter because she is a "helper." If the counselor then discovers that she really cannot become engaged in the client's subject matter, then the counselor may feel like a failure because she could not overcome her initial reluctance. Counselors need to assess where their interests lie and work with clients who match those interests assisting other clients by referring them to helpers who have an interest in their areas of need.

Case Study: Referral Due to Incompatibility of Interest Areas

> Beth was interested in and specialized in marriage counseling. She also was involved in family counseling but found long-term individual counseling uninteresting and unproductive. Beth had a referral from a very close friend, and felt that she had to take the client on as a favor to her long-time friend. Beth met with Jane for several sessions but found Jane's depression very difficult to deal with in the individual sessions. Beth preferred the structure and the interaction of marital couples. She found herself dreading Jane's sessions. Finally, Beth referred Jane to a therapist who specialized in depression. Jane received the referral willingly, sensing Beth's discomfort in working with her.

Sabotage of the Counseling Relationship

Clients enter counseling with hopes of positive change. However, even if a client is motivated to change, the actual change process can be difficult, painful, and exhausting. Counselors may encounter clients who resist attempts at bonding and intervention so that the counseling does not progress. Therapists will find that resistance occurs frequently with unmotivated and court-referred clients. Sabotage of the counseling relationship occurs because the client wants healthy change but does not want to make the painful discovery necessary for healing. He may show signs of resistance, he may have strong transference issues, or he may resent the fact that he has to be in counseling. He then may exhibit typical acting-out behavior, such as missing appointments, not paying for the sessions, not working on issues between sessions, refusing to talk, communicating about tangential subjects, or verbally attacking the therapist. The actions may vary but the message is the same. The client is saying that he does not want the counseling relationship to work and will undermine all attempts of the counselor to work with him.

Novice counselors often report feelings of having failed to engage such a client, forgetting that counseling is a two-way endeavor. Counselors cannot perform miracles and do not "cause" change. Clients are the change agents. Counselors need only to reverse the roles to see the error of their thinking. If the client were trying to engage the counselor in a relationship and the counselor was missing appointments, refusing to talk, communicating on tangential subjects, and verbally attacking the client, then would anyone expect therapeutic progress to occur?

Sabotage is easily recognized when the client exhibits overt acting-out behavior which leaves the counselor feeling frustrated, powerless, and, at times, angry. Sabotage is not as easily recognized when an unmotivated client participates in counseling sessions without working between sessions. These clients hang on month after month, remaining active during the sessions but making little progress. They may also allow minor conflicts to displace their counseling appointment. These clients evoke feelings of failure in their therapists because they appear to be cooperative or, at least, consistent in attending. Therapists therefore begin to blame themselves for the lack of progress. Such clients are often brought to the supervisory session in an attempt to find some technique or means to help the client. These clients would not mind if the counselor found a way to change them, as long as they do not have to do anything but attend the sessions. They are unwilling to expend the energy necessary to engage and maintain a relationship or effect change.

Recognizing these clients often brings immediate relief to the counselor and dissipates the feeling of failure. Further, recognition frees the counselor to consider referral or termination. Whether the client is sabotaging the relationship by acting out or by being unmotivated, the counselor should consider referral to a group as an alternative. Groups can help unmotivated or sabotaging clients through peer support and confrontation. Groups have an established track record for breaking through the tough resistance of reluctant clients.

GUILT

Guilt is a kindred emotion to failure. While failure denotes lack of success, guilt implies accountability and wrong doing. Many counseling relationships fail through no fault of the counselor. However, if a counselor feels guilty about the need to refer, she needs to ascertain what she actually did or did not do to make the referral necessary. Counselors pride themselves on their mental health, knowledge of people, ethical standards, and mastery of counseling theory and practice. However, helpers, being human, make mistakes and take responsibility for their errors in judgment.

Guilty feelings, although normal, are self-defeating. If a counselor must refer and has not erred in her treatment of the client, then guilt should not be a factor in this referral. If the counselor feels guilty during a routine referral, she needs to discover why. The issue for the counselor may be that the referral triggered a response to incidents much earlier in life when she was made to feel culpable for circumstances that were ordinary or routine.

However, if the counselor feels guilty about an action or omission in which she truly was accountable, then the feeling is justified and needs to be worked through so that the counselor can emerge from the experience with increased understanding and maturity.

Case Study #1: Guilt, Responsibility, and Referral

> Clara entered therapy with a counselor who was the director of the counseling center. Clara felt fragile as she began her therapeutic journey with her new counselor. She has just experienced an extremely volatile and unstable relationship. She felt rejected, was unsure of her future, and experienced identity confusion.
>
> Clara was struck, from the beginning of the therapeutic relationship, with Sally's patience. The therapeutic relationship developed over the first few months. Transference was strong as Clara worked on parental issues.

> However, during the middle phase of counseling, Clara began attending graduate school. A few months later Clara's graduate school required that she participate in an internship and Clara applied for an internship at Sally's counseling center. Clara was turned down with no reasons given for the rejection. However, Clara was offered a clerical job at the reception desk at the same center. After a month, Clara was given permission to see some of the clients. Therefore, Clara began seeing clients in the very center where she was a client. Then, half an hour before one of her sessions with Sally, Clara was informed by Sally that she was healthy and her counseling was therefore terminated. Clara was at a loss with no place to process her feelings. Clara did not want to terminate and was unsure about whether she was finished with her therapy. She was also somewhat mistrustful of starting another counseling relationship because of the enmeshment and rejection she had experienced.

While the ethical consideration of the dual role of employee/client is very apparent, the issue of referral is central to the successful resolution of this case. Clients occasionally seek employment, supervision, and/or education from their counselor or at their counselor's agency. Ethically, boundaries must be maintained and the client referred to another therapist outside the agency. In the above case, the client was allowed to hold a dual relationship with her counselor and agency. However, when the counselor finally did decide that the relationship was not ethical, no referral was discussed with the client. The client was instead left hanging, being told she was healthy, but feeling that she needed counseling and not free to say so for fear of losing her job. The counselor felt embarrassed because of her ethical mistake and so compounded it by terminating the client without processing. The client felt intimidated and insecure and plainly needed referral.

Sally continued to feel guilty about how she had muddied the waters by hiring Clara and then abruptly severed their therapeutic relationship. Sally had erred in her judgment twice regarding Clara, and had to take a close look at how she had reacted to the uncomfortable situation she had created. Sally began to see a pattern in her life whereby she confounds errors by additional errors. By exploring the dynamics of her mistake, Sally was able to transform her feeling of guilt into a catalyst for her own growth.

Case Study #2: Guilt, Responsibility, and Referral

> Bruce entered counseling hoping to increase his self-esteem. He had read a book that Ryan had written on the subject and decided that Ryan was the only counselor for him. Ryan interviewed Bruce and was flattered that Bruce had read his book. However, after a couple of sessions Ryan realized that he had made a mistake. Bruce did have self-esteem issues, but he was also an actively drinking alcoholic. Ryan knew that he had to refer Bruce to a detox unit, but when he imparted that information Bruce became enraged. Bruce denied his alcoholism and accused Ryan of being "just like the others." Bruce verbally berated Ryan for tricking him (writing an engaging book), getting him to collect his fee, and then rejecting (referring) him.
>
> Ryan felt guilty for beginning a relationship with Bruce. Ryan played "What if . . . " for weeks trying to assess what error in judgment he had committed. Finally, Ryan shared his experience at a case conference. The other counselors affirmed Ryan's actions and further questioned why Ryan was taking the responsibility for Bruce's decisions, assumptions, and drinking. Ryan explored his compulsion for being accountable for everything that happens in his life, especially in his counseling practice. When he began to realize that he expected to have control over others' reactions, Ryan was able to let go of his feeling of guilt over Bruce's abrupt termination and was able to let Bruce own his problems and their solutions or lack of solutions.

A counselor who is experiencing guilt can do the following to begin the process of assessment:

1. Determine what she did that was an error in judgment.
2. If there was no error, then the counselor should ask why she is feeling guilty. This can be accomplished through individual or group supervision, consultation, or personal therapy.

3. If the counselor does identify an error or mistake, then she needs to ask herself why it occurred and how it can be prevented in the future. Once again, supervision, consultation, and therapy can assist in sorting through the circumstances surrounding the problem.

4. Accept the problem as a learning and growing experience that she can draw on in the future to help others.

ANGER

Anger is a generalized emotional response that can yield feelings ranging from mild displeasure to overwhelming rage that borders on loss of control. Therapists feel angry more frequently than they express anger. Both therapists and clients have difficulty grappling with anger. Clients often report that they "should not" feel anger, especially at their parents, because anger is an unacceptable emotion. However, anger is an important feeling and should not be denied by client or counselor.

When a referral is necessary, a counselor may feel angry at the client, herself, the situation, or another who may be involved. Several different situations may result in anger at the client.

The Client Does Not Follow Through with the Therapeutic Contract

When a client and counselor enter the therapeutic contract, both assume responsibility to work toward a common goal of improved mental health for the client. The counselor pledges to be available during the client's scheduled therapeutic hour, to give the client her undivided attention, to use her skills and knowledge to help the client, to give honest feedback, and to maintain confidentiality. The client pledges to participate in the scheduled therapeutic hour; to honestly share his feelings, observations, and behavior; to process the session throughout the interim until the next session and to incorporate the changes discussed in counseling into his life outside the counseling arena.

If the counselor takes her pledge seriously and the client does not, then the counselor could experience anger at the client for not having held up his end of the contract. The anger may be expressed in terms of righteous indignation or resentment of the perceived wasted time. The counselor may need to refer and also feel anger at having to do so because she invested so much time and effort into the relationship, only to have the client decline the opportunity for change.

Case Study: Referral Due to Client's Lack of Follow-through

> Fred was referred to Irene by his gay lover after an accidental overdose. Fred expressed remorse at his error and said that he was extremely motivated to make changes in his lifestyle. Irene and Fred agreed to enter into a therapeutic contract. Irene spent many hours outside the counseling session reading and researching gay issues. Fred worked hard the first month, reporting that he was making progress with his counseling goals. However, Fred began abusing drugs and Irene was forced to make a referral to an inpatient setting.
>
> Irene was angry at Fred. He had broken the therapeutic contract and lost the potential of working on his problem without hospitalization. Fred expressed remorse and stated that he really felt that he had "blown it." Irene expressed her disappointment to Fred but refrained from saying she was angry out of concern that Fred would not return for any outpatient therapy after his hospitalization. However, at supervision, Irene was able to express her extreme anger at having to make the referral after having invested so much time and energy in understanding Fred.

The Client Sabotages the Counseling Relationship

The client's sabotage of the counseling relationship was addressed in the discussion of the counselor's feeling of failure. However, counselors can experience anger instead of failure when a client undermines the therapy.

Case Study: Anger at Client Sabotage

> Missy was referred to Sara by her school counselor. Missy was truant from school, complained about her parents' neglect of her, and exhibited depression. Missy's parents supported her counseling, but Missy was ambivalent. However, Missy and Sara did begin to bond well. Missy was very grateful to have someone to talk to about all of her feelings about her parents. Sara listened well and empathized with Missy's situation. However, after several sessions, Missy decided to express her negative feelings to her parents. Missy began by telling her parents how she felt about them but after receiving a hostile reaction, Missy claimed that Sara had put all the negative ideas in her head. Missy's parents were very angry and came to Missy's next session. Sara was able to straighten out the miscommunication, and recommended that the whole family enter family counseling. They agreed, so Sara made the referral. Sara was very angry at Missy and knew that a referral was necessary because the trust between them had broken down when Missy sabotaged the counseling. Sara felt righteous indignation and let Missy know how she felt. While Sara felt better for having vented her anger, she regretted expressing her anger to her client because she knew that Missy would now see her as simply another critical parent.

The Client Shows Extreme Resistance

Resistance is the reluctance of the client to participate in the very activity which he knows will bring about positive change. Resistance is therefore self-defeating for the client. Most clients show signs of resistance at some point in the therapeutic process. However, some clients are resistant from the moment they enter counseling. Resistance can be exhibited by many different behaviors. Helpers who encounter forms of resistance often consider referral as an option as they express anger toward the client. Week after week, resistant clients take up the counselor's time with no-shows, excuses, hostile interactions, no movement, and irrelevant communication. Frequently, counselors may become angry and frustrated enough to consider termination without referral. However, referral can work for these clients if they are carefully connected with the appropriate counselor or group.

Referral of the extremely resistant client can be a positive therapeutic experience if the counselor:

1. Models appropriate expression of her anger and disappointment in the client's lack of cooperation;
2. Lets the client know that the therapeutic relationship is valuable and worth taking seriously;
3. Confronts the resistance directly by asking the client why he does not want to participate in therapy;
4. Selects a new counselor with a strong track record in working with resistant clients;
5. Selects a group that has a positive reputation for working with resistant clients.

Case Study: Anger at Client Resistance

Michele started seeing Peter because she was being repeatedly battered by her alcoholic husband. Michele had a dependent personality disorder and talked about her problem with her mother and her sister routinely. Michele asked Peter to help her become strong enough to leave her husband, Joe. Each week, Peter and Michele worked on Michele's dependency. Peter gave Michele several phone numbers of shelters to call if she was being threatened by Joe. Each week, Michele saw Peter and reported repetitive physical abuse, but she never called a shelter. Peter began to experience anger at Michele and started thinking about referral to a women's support group and a female therapist who specialized in spouse abuse. Michele also told Peter that she had packed her bags many times, only to be talked out of leaving by her mother and sister who told Michele that she would be committing a sin if she left her husband. Peter found himself getting angry at Michele's mother and sister. He even tried having them in for a session. Peter reported being totally frustrated, fearful for Michele's safety, and angry at Michele and her family, as well as infuriated at himself for dragging his feet on the referral.

Peter finally referred Michele, much to Michele's disappointment. Through the group, Michele received much-needed peer support. The female therapist was able to encourage transference, which was necessary for Michele to work through her dependency on her mother. By contrast, Michele had seen Peter as "the good husband" for whom she felt she had to appear the helpless victim.

Peter never expressed his anger to Michele or her family, but he did talk about his feelings with his supervisor. Because of his anger, Peter had missed the transference that was supporting the unhealthy system. As he accepted and expressed his anger, Peter became aware of how a counselor's emotions can cloud the objective view of the client.

FEAR

When a counselor must refer a client to another helper, she may experience fear or anxiety in several areas. A counselor may be afraid that the referral source or her colleagues will see her as inept or inexperienced because she had to make a referral. She may be afraid or concerned that the client will not follow through with the referral. She may feel apprehensive about whether the new counselor will view her work with the client an incompetent or unskilled. She may be anxious that she is not completing the referral process correctly. Finally, she may be afraid of referring the client to the wrong counselor.

Making a therapeutic referral is a serious responsibility involving more than simply handing the client a new counselor's name. It is, therefore, understandable if the counselor experiences fear or at least anxiety over the outcome of her referral efforts. However, helpers need not allow their fear or anxiety to interfere with their obligation to make the referral a positive therapeutic process. Discussions of the above four concerns elsewhere in this book offer guidelines to help overcome counselor's fear and uncertainty due to inexperience or performance anxiety.

REJECTION

When a client suggests the referral or eagerly accepts a referral, the counselor can experience feelings of surprise, failure, and rejection. Counselors are especially vulnerable to rejection when they believe that they have built a positive therapeutic relationship with the client, when they have worked hard at the client's problem, or when they are susceptible to rejection because of their own therapeutic issues. Before addressing each of these possible reasons for feelings of rejection, a word of caution is necessary. Clients will usually not ask for a referral when they want to leave therapy. More often, they will terminate the therapeutic relationship when they believe that the therapy is not working or is not for them. Then, after termination, they may seek another counselor. If counselors feel rejected when the client asks for a referral or terminates prematurely, the problem can be that the counselor is not able to make a therapeutic referral because she is too busy feeling hurt, rejected, or angry to pay attention to her client's needs. The professional helper has a responsibility to put her feelings aside in order to assist the client with his referral and then to work through the feelings caused by the perceived rejection.

Even if a helper perceives that the relationship with the client is progressing and has worked hard at the client's problems, the client may experience the situation differently. For example, the client may not be bonding therapeutically because he may be sexually attracted to his therapist, he may feel overwhelmed by the therapeutic issues confronting him, he may feel threatened by the intimacy of the therapeutic relationship, he may not have developed trust in his counselor, or he may feel that he needs a different type of counselor. Therefore, the therapist must put her feelings of rejection on hold and explore the client's desire for termination or referral. Helping the client to identify his reasons and emotions about wanting to leave counseling or wanting another counselor will serve two purposes. First, the discussion will help the client to clarify his ideas and feelings so that he will be better prepared to enter his next counseling relationship. Second, the discussion will shed some light on the reasons for the referral/termination request of the client. If the counselor can learn more about the client's feelings, the counselor may not need to feel rejected by the client, and will be better able to make an appropriate referral on behalf of the client.

Since it is possible that the counselor may feel positive about the helping relationship and the client may not, the counselor may feel rejected. This does not necessarily mean that the client is rejecting the helper, only the counselor's help. Counselors need to emphasize this difference. Questions such as the following may help the therapist to work on her feelings of rejection:

1. Has the counselor's experience been that most of her clients reject her help?
2. Has the counselor received any criticism from her supervisors or teachers that she has ignored?
3. Has the counselor received feedback from clients or peers that she would rather not hear and has therefore ignored?
4. Has the counselor experienced rejection in her past that has not been resolved and could therefore be exacerbating the feelings connected with the client's rejection of her?
5. Does the counselor use denial frequently to delude herself into thinking that everything is going well, causing her to ignore critical clues that other are sending?
6. Does the counselor work well with certain types of clients but insist on taking clients who should be referred to counselors with different theoretical styles?

Clients who reject their therapist's help can evoke feelings of hurt, anger, or confusion in the therapist. The therapist may defend against these feelings by denial, projection, or intellectualization. However, counselors who are willing to explore their own feelings as well as those of their clients, will be in a better position to make the client-initiated referral a therapeutic process.

GRIEVING

Whenever a relationship or a potential relationship is lost, there is the possibility of grieving. In the case of referral, a counselor's feeling of loss would depend on the reason for the referral and what the counselor feels about giving up the counseling relationship with the client.

If the client is being referred for being resistant, or combative, or for sabotaging the counseling, then the counselor may not experience grief at all. In fact, the counselor may feel relief about the loss of the client. At other times, the counselor may feel neutral about the referral. This might occur when the relationship did not gel, the counselor referred the client shortly after the initial contact, or the counselor was not strongly invested in the relationship. However, if the client has bonded well, worked hard, and progressed toward health, then the counselor may experience a sense of grief over the loss of the working relationship. Counselors often neglect this feeling and suppose that it is unprofessional to have feelings of positive attachment toward a client. Denying the feelings and acting aloof or unconcerned does not cause the feelings to disappear. Nor does the counselor's denial assist the client with his referral process. In fact, the client may feel rejected and unaffirmed by a counselor who uses defenses instead of confronting the emotions that she is currently experiencing.

Case Study: Grieving and Referral

> Charles saw Delores for three months before referring her to another therapist because he had decided to take a full-time position as an Employee Assistance Program specialist. Delores accepted the referral but expressed her positive feelings for Charles as the one person who had made a difference in her

life. Charles was feeling very sad about ending the therapeutic relationship with Delores. He had developed an admiration for Delores and her progress with her struggle. Charles's grief at having to refer Delores took an extreme form. He set up extra sessions with Delores on the pretense of getting her to a different level of health before referring her; he became angry at the referral resource for not returning Delores's telephone call immediately; he tried bargaining with his soon-to-be-past employer for office space so that he might continue to see Delores, and he regretted losing her as a client. Charles's supervisor told him that his grieving was unhealthy, causing his actions to become unprofessional. He recommended that Charles become more professional in his dealing with Delores. Charles then became distant and analytical with Delores. She felt betrayed and angry, accusing Charles of caring for her only because she was paying him. When Delores changed therapists, she had to spend many sessions working through the betrayal she felt and rebuilding trust in the therapeutic process.

Charles concluded that he had misunderstood his supervisor's advice to be more professional with Delores. As he worked on his feelings in his personal counseling, Charles came to realize that his feelings of grief were not the problem. He understood that his grieving over the loss of the relationship was totally normal, and that it was his actions that were the problem.

If Charles had accepted his feelings as normal and healthy, then he would not have felt the need to reject Delores as he did. Instead, he could have explored his grieving, appreciated his relationship with Delores, and wished Delores good luck in her next therapeutic relationship. Delores would have benefitted from Charles's openness and continued concern for her and would have been able to participate in her next counseling relationship without having to spend weeks dealing with the negative referral experience.

When a counselor must refer a client and they both are experiencing grief over the loss, the counselor might postpone termination with the client despite having made a referral. While this continuation activity may appear to be a weaning of the client from the referring counselor, it can delay or exacerbate the grieving process while interfering with the new counselor's ability to establish a trusting counseling relationship. Further, the postponement interferes with the client's therapy if the two therapists are working on different issues. While the pain of separation and loss is great, the most therapeutic behavior is to refer the client appropriately, to spend a session reminiscing and saying goodbye and to let go of the client so that he can form a new therapeutic alliance.

CONCLUSION

Helpers are not immune from feelings concerning the referral of clients. It is extremely important for counselors and other helpers who are involved in referring clients to recognize their affective state as normal, to accept their emotions, to explore the countertransference issues which may arise, and to ensure that their own feelings do not interfere in the process of the therapeutic referral.

6

Approaching the Client About the Referral

The initial approach to the client about the prospect of referral must be handled appropriately so that the client does not feel that he is being rejected by his counselor. Also, it is important to avoid giving the client the impression that he needs a higher powered therapist because he is too dysfunctional for his current helper to handle (Downing, 1985). In some instances where the referral is being made by a minister, school counselor, or other helper who may not be trained or able to work with clients on a long-term basis, the helper's tendency may be openly to emphasize and admit her limitations, thus revealing to the client that he has very difficult problems that require a more highly trained helper. The referring helper may actually believe this to be the case, and may believe that her honesty with the client is the best policy. However, the therapeutic procedure is for the referring helper to approach the client with an attitude of desiring to match the client with the helper who is most congruent with the client's need and problem areas.

A client who deliberately makes his initial contact with a helper who is not in a position to develop a weekly therapeutic relationship (such as a pastor, or school counselor) may be testing the waters to see if a more objective person thinks that he needs help. If that same helper reacts with an attitude of "You need more help than I can give you," then the client can feel rejected, scared, and overwhelmed with the apprehension that his worst fears are realized.

The manner of introducing the subject of referral to the client will vary depending upon the stage of intervention in which the present helping relationship is functioning.

REFERRAL AT THE INITIAL STAGE OF COUNSELING

When a prospective client approaches a helper for an initial consultation, he may be wanting some advice as to whether he should seek counseling, he may wish to talk to someone briefly, he may be looking for long-term help, or he may be looking for a referral.

At this initial stage, the helper could be someone the prospective client knows and trusts, such as his teacher, pastor, or guidance counselor, or she may be a total stranger to whom the client risks talking about his problem. No matter what the degree or extent of the relationship, the helper has a major responsibility to assess the client's situation and decide whether and to whom the client needs to be referred and how to approach the client about needing referral.

While meeting with the prospective client, student, parishioner, or acquaintance, the helper can do the following to enable the referral process:

1. Listen carefully and actively to what and how the client is communicating. From this information, the referring helper can arrive at a tentative diagnosis ascertaining the type of helper that will be best suited to assist the client.
2. Support the client in his desire to get help for his presenting problem.
3. Help the client to identify the specific problems with which he desires help.

4. Help the client to identify the ways in which he can begin to address his problems. This discussion will ultimately lead to talking about a type of therapeutic intervention. It is at this point that the helper can decide to offer to see the client, if appropriate, or to suggest a referral.

5. Be aware of the possibility that the client may view referral as a statement of the great severity of his problem.

6. If the helper has chosen referral, then she should let the client know why she is recommending referral, that the referral resource being considered is skilled in the treatment of the client's problem, and that she will scrvc as a bridge between the client and the referral resource.

7. Affirm the client's wisdom in seeking help with his problems.

8. In letting the client know why the helper has chosen to refer, avoid using language that could lead the client to feel unwanted, rejected, or "unhelpable" (Ritchie, 88). Instead the helper should emphasize that the reason for referral is based on the client's best interest and not because:
   a. the client has problems that are severe and overwhelming to most counselors;
   b. the helper is unable or unwilling to assist the client;
   c. the helper does not care;
   d. the client is scaring the helper.

9. Allow the client time to process the information he has just shared and received.

10. Remember that although the helper is acting therapeutically, the helper is not the client's counselor during this stage. The helper should not focus on insight, background, therapeutic homework, intervention, or transference. The helper should focus on what the problem is, how it affects the client's life, what the client is prepared to do about his problem, the best course of action for the client, and the best provider of therapeutic service.

11. The client and helper should approach the referral as a cooperative search for the optimal provider of therapeutic services for the client.

Once the client has had some time to process the information that he has received, he will be ready to make a commitment to the counseling referral. Some clients need very little time, others may think about the referral for weeks or months, while others may choose not to follow through at all. While the client who quickly decides to accept the referral is the most desirable client, the helper needs to understand that the time taken for communication with the prospective client is not wasted if the client does not follow through in a reasonable time. The helper may have tilled the soil for further work; however, the client may not take advantage of counseling for years.

If the client has accepted referral, then the counselor can begin the process of preparing the client for the actual process of referral. This process is discussed later in this chapter.

REFERRAL AT THE MIDDLE STAGE OF COUNSELING

The reasons why counselors refer after the therapeutic relationship has begun have been discussed earlier in this book. The key question to ask at this time is whether the current therapeutic relationship is more important to the progress of the client than referral. Interrupting the therapeutic process to refer a client calls for careful deliberation and consultation with the therapist's supervisor. It is critical to take into account the client's feelings, needs, and progress to date before committing to referral.

If it is determined that referral is necessary during the middle phase of counseling, it must be approached with special attention since the therapeutic alliance is so well developed. The helper must allow time to process, time to grieve, and time to share feelings. In addition, the communication style must be gentle, accepting, direct, firm, and nonthreatening. In many instances, the client has just begun to open up wounds and address concerns that he may have long ignored. In this raw state, referral is not desirable. So when it is *necessary,* care must be taken to approach the subject carefully and to spend the time necessary to make the referral therapeutic.

Here-and-Now Issues in the Counseling Relationship

The counselor should begin by sharing with the client her understanding of what is happening in the counseling relationship at present (here-and-now). If the counselor feels that bonding has not occurred, then the client and counselor need to process this together. Another here-and-now issue is resistance. A client who demonstrates massive resistance may not be consciously aware of what is occurring and a discussion about what is happening may assist the client in overcoming the resistance. Focusing on the here and now will also assist the counselor to stay on the subject of referral and not become involved with what has occurred in the client's past, which is best left to the referral resource to handle.

Lack of Skills

A counselor may feel positive about having developed a counseling relationship with the client only to discover in the middle of working with the client that the client is presenting new problems that the counselor believes she is not skilled enough to handle. The counselor needs to approach the client about receiving help from a different source without letting him know that she is feeling unskilled in dealing with the problem. This is important for two reasons. First, this revelation may lead the client to feel that he has more severe problems than he does. He may jump to the conclusion that since the person he has trusted and under whom he has progress cannot help him, then he surely must be very dysfunctional. Second, the client can feel that his counselor has been duping him about her skill level. He may feel betrayed and believe that the counselor was only keeping him as a client for the fees he paid.

Counselors pride themselves on being open and honest in their dealings with their clients and may feel uncomfortable in not sharing all their honest shortcomings with their client at the time of referral. However, referring a client because the counselor feels that her skill level is not as strong as another counselor's and wants the best for her client does not mean that the referring counselor is

unskilled. The client who is being referred may not be able to hear the difference, or may be experiencing emotions that distort what the counselor is saying about her lack of skills.

The counselor can better assist the client with the referral process by approaching the subject positively, with deep care and concern for the client, as illustrated in the case study that follows.

Case Study: Approaching the Client

Karyn started seeing Mark in a pastoral counseling setting because she was experiencing panic attacks, a poor marital relationship, and job difficulties. Karyn saw Mark for nine months, during which time Mark taught Karyn relaxation techniques. They also worked on Karyn's job difficulties and her feelings about marriage. After nine months, Karyn began remembering horrible, mutilating child abuse scenes from her past. Mark felt that he was not the best person to deal with Karyn's unresolved childhood pain, even though he felt that he and Karyn had a very positive therapeutic relationship. He also felt very unskilled in dealing with the horrendous scenes that Karyn was describing. Mark decided referral was necessary and planned his approach with the help of his supervisor:

1. Mark summarized the progress that they had made so far based on Karyn's presenting problems. Karyn agreed that she felt stronger than she ever had before and she believed that it was because she was stronger that her memory was returning.
2. Mark agreed that she was strong enough to face the truth from the past and that was why her early childhood memory was free to return.
3. Mark told Karyn that she was entering a new and different therapeutic stage which required very specific skills.
4. Mark also told Karyn that she deserved to see a therapist who had been trained to work with the healing of early childhood memories. Karyn agreed but began to express concern over not seeing mark, since she trusted him.
5. Mark appreciated Karyn's comments and told her that he cared for her and wanted to see her healthy as expediently as

possible. He told Karyn that if she did trust him that she needed to trust him with this referral. Karyn hesitantly agreed to see the new therapist.

6. Mark invited the new therapist, Beverly, to join him and Karyn in a session. Karyn bonded with Beverly and they all agreed that Karyn should continue in one of Mark's groups.

7. When Beverly and Karyn finished their work together, Beverly suggested that Karyn and her husband see Mark for marriage counseling, one of Mark's specialties. Karyn's husband was so impressed with Mark's handling of Karyn's problems and referral, that he was totally trusting of Mark's skills although Mark had a previous therapeutic relationship with Karyn.

The above case is an ideal situation, but it is a real story. The referral process did occur as outlined above and shows that a counselor need not confess his lack of skills blatantly in order to assist in a referral. Mark used a very positive approach and thereby lost no credibility and did not denigrate his skill level. Karyn's return to Mark with her husband for marriage counseling bears this out.

Countertransference

When a client has evoked countertransference responses from the counselor and the counselor decides she must refer the client to another helper, the therapist needs to approach the subject of referral carefully. Every counselor will have countertransference issues at some time in her career, and should be prepared for this eventuality.

Clients have a need to see their therapist as psychologically healthier than themselves. Clients have a difficult time seeing their therapists as human beings with typical emotions, past issues, and current problems. Rather, clients tend to see their therapists as "having it all together." Therefore, sharing all the countertransference details, reasons, and issues with the client may harm the therapeutic relationship and future therapeutic relationships.

First, the client needs to have confidence in the present relationship and the progress that he has made. An explanation of countertransference and the therapist's unresolved issues toward the client could discount the progress made in therapy to date. Second, a client who needs to be referred may lose confidence in the therapeutic process if he is told that his counselor is experiencing countertransference with him. Third, some clients may try to precipitate another countertransference reaction in their next therapist in an attempt to sabotage their counseling. Confessing countertransference issues to such a client reinforces his belief that he can manipulate even intelligent, skilled helpers. Fourth, if a counselor wants to make a therapeutic referral, the counselor must be credible to the client. If the client loses respect for or confidence in the counselor, he may lose confidences in the referral process or the helping process.

Therefore, in dealing with referral due to unresolved countertransference the counselor should approach the client in much the same way she would if she were referring a client because she felt that her skills were not sufficient.

1. Affirm the therapeutic relationship.
2. Affirm the progress that the client has made while in counseling.
3. Explain that the client is at a point in his growth which requires a therapeutic alliance different from yours.
4. If the client objects and asserts that he really needs and trusts the present counselor, be affirming and caring, and explain that you cannot be as therapeutic with the client given the subject matter of his current problems.
5. Emphasize that the decision took a great deal of careful thought and considerable time and was not an easy one to make, but was based on what was best for the client.
6. Assure the client that he is not being rejected or blamed for the need to refer.
7. Assert that, as the referring counselor, you are committed to cooperatively assisting the client in connecting with a counselor with whom he will be able to address his problems.
8. Remain firm, calm; and affirming in the face of the client's pleading, grieving, anger, and accusations.

9. Seek therapeutic help in working with the countertransference issues.

10. Make the referral (see other chapters for this process).

Irreconcilable Logistical Problems

There are many reasons why the counselor and client may be unable to continue meeting: counselor takes another job, client or counselor is moving, client takes a job that conflicts with availability of counselor, client or counselor becomes physically ill. Although these reasons for referral seem straightforward and understandable, emotions can still play a part in making the referral difficult. Both client and counselor may agree that there are no alternatives to referral and still not feel comfortable with the solution. Approaching the client in the middle phase of counseling about an inevitable referral requires as much tact and affirmation as when there are countertransference issues. The client may accept the undeniable reason for referral and still need to grieve over the loss of his therapist whom he has depended on and with whom he has begun to experience health. The tendency is to rush the referral which is clearly needed because of the irreconcilable logistical problems. However, this referral needs the same careful processing as any other.

1. Establish with the client that there is no other way to meet his therapeutic need except through referral. This takes more time than is usually expected. The client and the counselor may experience denial so that a period of brainstorming on how they can overcome the logistical problem may emerge. Clients may have to entertain the most bizarre solutions only to discard them in order to arrive at acceptance. Let this process take place without rushing it. Who knows; the client may actually find a way!

2. Once referral is established as the only way to meet the therapeutic needs of the client, allow time for the grieving of both client and counselor. Explore the anger at external events that caused this interruption of the helping relationship. Accept the bargaining and depression as normal.

3. Share your feelings of grief with the client.
4. Assure the client that the job of referral is another method of helping the client.
5. Dedicate as much energy to arriving at a cooperative choice of the new therapist as was needed to work on the client's therapeutic issues.
6. Affirm the progress that has been made so far.
7. With the client, identify the therapeutic issues remaining to be addressed.
8. Connect the client with the new therapist. (see other chapters for this process).

It is important not to hurry through this separation process. Allow time for both of you to experience grief and to work toward the connection with the referral resource. Terminating too abruptly may evoke feelings of rejection or abandonment which may prevent the client from following through.

Networking

There will be times when a helper may need to network with other helpers to provide the client with a holistic therapeutic experience, while still maintaining the primary responsibility for the client's therapy. Clients may see this as an attempt by the therapist to disengage from her responsibility, or as an admission that she cannot help her client without others' assistance. Other clients may view the networking as an indication that they really do need a lot more help. Counselors may not recognize that these clients' feelings of abandonment, rejection, and betrayal are so strong that they take the most innocent helping network as a threat. Therefore, it is important to approach any networking decision as carefully as one would approach a referral:

1. Explain to the client that there are many ways of obtaining health and that you want to offer as many opportunities as possible to the client.
2. Assure the client that the networking opportunity in no way

means that the therapy is being transferred. Assure him that this is a broadening of the counseling scope not a substitution.

3. Share as much knowledge as possible about the network opportunity. If the referral is for medication, testing, or evaluation, reassure the client that these are only possibilities and that ultimately the client has the responsibility to decide whether he will accept the medication or recommendation. (For noncompliant clients, see section later in this chapter.)

4. Approach the networking positively, emphasizing that the client will learn more about himself.

5. Affirm that any decisions to be made can be discussed during the counseling sessions.

6. Emphasize the evaluative and educative possibilities of networking.

7. Affirm the progress that has been made and show how the network can contribute to the client's further progress.

8. Above all, approach the entire subject in an upbeat nonthreatening, enthusiastic manner that evokes trust, curiosity, and confidence. The key words are "opportunity to learn."

There will also be times when the counselor wants the client to take advantage of a group experience while still being involved in individual counseling. While some clients may be interested in supplementing their therapy with group counseling, some clients may feel seriously threatened by the though of either a group experience or seeing another therapist in group. Group processes complement individual counseling well. This is especially true for co-dependent family members of alcoholics, those experiencing grief, recovering alcoholics and drug addicts, those with eating disorders, adult survivors of childhood sexual abuse, and rape victims. In order to gain the client's cooperation and interest in taking part in a group:

1. Approach the subject of group by pointing out that many others share feelings and problems similar to those of the client. Clients may volunteer at this point that they do not know of anyone else who is struggling with their issue.

2. Mention to the client that there are groups at which he may meet others who are being challenged by the same issues; and suggest that he may want to take the opportunity to join such a group.

3. Outline gently (no hard sell) the benefits of group work and how it can supplement the individual work which the client is now doing. Emphasize that one type of counseling is not a substitute for the other.

4. During this dialogue, the matter of fees will probably arise. Some clients have difficulty in paying for their individual sessions. To add a group on top of their already difficult financial outlay may be more than they can afford. Counselors have found several solutions to the problem.

   a. The client can wait to take advantage of the group until he is ready to terminate individual therapy.
   b. The counselor can reduce her fee to allow the client the possibility of participation.
   c. If the therapist is collecting insurance, then often insurance will pay for the group.
   d. The counselor can find a low-fee or free group, if one exists.
   e. The counselor can find a sliding scale group which may be less expensive for the client.
   f. The counselor can suspend counseling for a brief period of time while the client participates in the group.
   g. The counselor can ask the client to re-evaluate his priorities to see if he could afford the group if he gave up something else. (For example, the client may give up smoking and use the money for the group.)

5. Affirm the work that the client has accomplished so far and explain how a group can augment the success.

6. Emphasize to the client that he lives in a world of groups and subgroups and that participation in a therapy group can assist him in his functioning in other areas of his life.

REFERRAL AT THE TERMINATION STAGE OF COUNSELING

When a client is approaching termination, he often feels a great sense of accomplishment but also a feeling of not wanting to let go of a relationship that has made a major difference in his life. Clients may need a bridge between the intensive work they are used to and being completely free of counseling. At this point, counselors may want to suggest a group experience, an educational workshop, family counseling, or marital counseling.

The last two are not to be confused with those instances where the family unit or marital unit is the client and where the primary therapeutic process is with the family or marital couple. (In these cases the family may refer an individual member for counseling upon termination.) It is important to recognize that when an individual changes, his family or marital unit may need some help in adjusting to the difference. Family and marital counseling can be extremely beneficial in these instances.

Case Study: Referral Upon Termination

> Dick started seeing Jim because of Dick's depression and poor self-image. Dick and Jim worked for eighteen months, at which time they began discussing termination. They both experienced a wonderful feeling of achievement, but Dick was especially worried about being cast adrift with no lifeline. In addition, Dick was questioning whether his current career was the correct one for him. Therefore, Jim suggested a competent career counselor and Dick met with the career counselor for two months and then returned to Jim to integrate what he had learned. Dick asked Jim about an on-going group to help him to process day-to-day problems and also receive some support. Jim referred Dick to a group with which Dick stayed connected for about nine months. Dick left the group feeling strong enough to face life without any therapeutic support.

Notice that although Jim had terminated his therapeutic relationship with Dick, Jim continued to act as the referral source for

Dick. Dick knew and trusted Jim's knowledge and connections to other helpers and used him as a referral source as he orchestrated his own health.

Approaching the terminating client who has had success in therapy with the idea of referral is fairly routine. The client is healthy and able to sort through whether he feels the need for further work. However, the client who is terminating against his therapist's advice will resist referral to any other therapy. Counselors need to be firm and confrontational in most cases. Sometimes the client takes a flight into health and pronounces himself better. At other times, that client may terminate prematurely because he has decided that he does not want to be in counseling and make changes. When this happens, the tendency is for the counselor to respect the client's choice and let the client leave after having stated that she disagrees with the client's choice. However, there are instances where the counselor can make an effective referral when a client decides to terminate prematurely.

When a client decides to terminate, he will usually tell the counselor that the counseling is not working for him and he feels it is a waste of time. The client may even say that the counselor has not helped him. The counselor can take this opportunity to talk about expectations concerning what counseling does and does not do. Few clients understand that the therapist is not going to be a change agent. Bringing this to the client's attention places the responsibility for the counseling where it belongs, on the client. Further, the counselor can tell the client that if the counseling relationship has not worked to the client's satisfaction, then the next step is for the counselor to make a referral to another helper with whom the client can have the chance to form a better therapeutic relationship. This offer:

1. Lets the client see the nondefensive stance of a counselor who has been unfairly accused of not working.
2. Lets the client hear that the counselor's main concern is the client's health.
3. Lets the client know that the therapeutic alliance is of prime concern and the client needs to participate in the relationship if it is to work.

4. Lets the client know that there may be another counselor with whom he can form a working alliance.

All this adds up to the possibility that the client may accept the referral when offered. Of course, the client may not accept the referral, or may pretend to accept the referral with no intention of following through. However, even if the client terminates prematurely and does not follow through, the client leaves the counselor's office with a better understanding of the counseling relationship and with the name of a counseling referral.

If the client makes a flight into health and justifies his termination because he is feeling better, then the counselor still has a responsibility to the client to let him know what she sees as his continuing problem. The counselor should also respect the client's need to see himself as healthy. However, the client can leave the counselor's office with a variety of referral or networking possibilities which he can take advantage of at any time.

TALKING ABOUT REFERRAL WITH VARIOUS CLIENTS

Different clients need to be approached in differing ways about referral. Although the previous pages reflect a conservative, supportive process of talking with clients about referral, each client engages in communication with different intensity depending on his style of interaction. For example, some clients want straight talk from their counselors. They want no roundabout communication. They appreciate honesty and would respect the counselor if she were to use self-disclosure. These clients tend to rush through the affective part of the referral in order to get on with the process. Counselors should help these clients by drawing their attention to the relationship and the grieving process. Also, knowing these clients well permits the counselors to be confrontational and direct.

Clients who operate out of the defensive posture of denial are particularly frustrating to deal with. They tend to not hear what they do not wish to hear and may even distort the rest. Although honest, straight talk seems to be the best way to probe through their denial, the fact is that they use denial when they feel the least bit threatened. Therefore, the better communication style is a non-threatening, calm, affirming posture where the client has time to slowly hear the referral and accept it.

Other clients use manipulation as a means to control their environment. Referring these clients will meet with resistance in the form of manipulation, which must be met with direct, honest communication. However, while using straight talk, the counselor may feel the need to push the client toward acceptance too quickly. Clients who manipulate try to make their environment meet their needs. Therefore, if they do not wish to be referred, they use every tactic they know to affect a change in the counselor's decision. They may precipitate a crisis, threaten suicide, become hostile and attack the counselor. These manipulations must be confronted in a gentle but firm manner. In addition to dealing with the manipulative communication style, the counselor must also encourage the client to accept his feelings, express his feelings in a nonmanipulative manner, and grieve the loss of the relationship. Using the previously presented material, the counselor should present the referral in the most direct but affirming manner possible. While it is important for the counselor to avoid being manipulated by the client, she must also maintain her patience with the client.

Another client who appreciates direct, honest communication is the client who has a positive relationship with his counselor. He trusts her and wants to feel that she would be truthful with him. For many clients, the counseling relationship is the first truly intimate, open, and honest relationship they have ever had. For these clients, the counselor must be quite honest about the referral and the impending process.

Some clients, however, are very fragile and are afraid to hear the truth except in very small doses. They are timid, dependent people who are afraid of others, of life, and of their own emotions. They usually expect to be rejected, abandoned, or betrayed and look for those experiences in every situation. These clients need to be approached cautiously about referral because they will sense rejection. The counselor must begin by asking questions that will lead the client into exploring the referral process. It is critical for the counselor to approach the subject of referral in such a way that the client feels he is being heard, that his best interest is at the heart of the decision, and that he has nothing to fear. Even so, the fragile client benefits from having the new referral resource join one of his sessions to assuage his fears and concerns.

WHAT NOT TO SAY OR DO WHEN INTRODUCING THE SUBJECT OF REFERRAL

While this chapter focuses on the most positive manner of approaching clients about referral, there are several behaviors or attitudes which must not be communicated to the client.

1. *Do not make assumptions.* When making a referral, one of the most common mistakes a counselor makes is to assume that she knows how the client is going to react to the news of referral because she has observed the client and assessed his typical reactions. Allow the client his own reaction and respond to that. Do not assume that the client will automatically follow through with the referral. Even the most motivated client can become disillusioned or apprehensive about the change of counselors, causing him to rethink his commitment to the referral.

2. *Do not make value judgments.* Words such as *better, worse, good, bad* can create a judgmental climate. A client needs to hear his helper discuss his referral in a positive, consistent process in which the client receives logical reasons and is encouraged to work on his feelings. The helper should avoid making judgments about the client's previous counseling experience, the client's reasons for not wanting referral, or the reason for the client to choose one referral resource over another.

Case Study: Referral and the Client's Choice of Therapist

> Debi, a high school guidance counselor, had spent a great deal of time with Fred, a senior at her high school. She realized that

> she was going to have to refer Fred because he needed long-term counseling which was outside her job description and time commitment to the school. When Debi mentioned to Fred that he needed to see someone regularly, Fred agreed but insisted that he go back to his former therapist, whom he had seen three years previously. Debi knew the therapist and did not hold him in high esteem. In fact, Debi questioned the therapist's ethical behavior with his clients. Debi felt an obligation to steer Fred toward another therapist even though she knew that Fred was loyal to his previous therapist. Debi approached the subject of seeing another therapist with Fred. She told Fred that although he might have enjoyed a positive relationship with his previous therapist three years ago, another counselor might be *better* able to help Fred today. Fred picked up on Debi's use of the word *better* and became angry at Debi for what he perceived as a put-down of his previous therapist. Debi recovered from the attack and realized that her feelings about Fred's previous therapist had infiltrated her manner of speaking about the therapist. Debi calmly told Fred that she had used a poor choice of words. She then told Fred that he could, of course, return to his previous therapist but that there were some excellent helpers near the school who were specially trained in treating his type of problem. Debi asked Fred to consider interviewing a couple of therapists so that he could make a decision based on his interactions with several different counselors. Fred did see two other counselors, but announced to Debi that he still felt more comfortable with his previous therapist so he returned to him for counseling. However, because Fred was three years older, he began to pick up on the previous therapist's lack of professionalism. He ceased seeing him and entered counseling with one of the two therapists whom he had interviewed three months earlier.

Counselors are trained to avoid judgmental words such as *better, should, worse*. However, when a referral is imminent and clients have several choices to make, the counselor can become enmeshed in the decision and show her prejudice toward one of the referral therapists. While clients need all the information that is necessary to make a decision, the therapist needs to allow the client the freedom to make the decision himself, even if the therapist disagrees with the decision.

3. *Do not oversell the referral resource.* There is a tendency when making a referral to encourage the client to follow through with the referral by building up the positive qualities of the new therapist. While the client does need to feel confident that he is being connected with an excellent referral resource, the client could begin to put his new therapist on a pedestal, which might interfere with the development of the therapeutic relationship. There is a fine line between giving the client an honest, positive appraisal of the prospective counselor and overappraising the work of the counselor so the client is set up to expect perfection. The best alternative is to state briefly the counselor's positive attributes and to emphasize that the referring helper holds the counselor in highest esteem. It is also wise to state that while there is no guarantee that the client and counselor will be able to establish a positive therapeutic relationship, a great deal of thought went into making the referral. Also the referring helper can offer to make another referral if the current one does not work out.

Another danger of overselling the new counselor is that the client may blame himself if the referral does not work. The client will see the counselor as nearing perfection, and so feel that the failed referral must be his fault. The client may conclude that he is not capable of being helped and may not seek further counseling.

4. *Do not undermine the current helping relationship or process.* A helper who feels overwhelmed by one of her parishioners, students, or patients and who wants to refer that person, may try to prove to her client that the current relationship is a poor substitute for a "real" therapeutic relationship. Ministers are particularly prone to this type of denigration. They often say, "I'm only your pastor." "I'm not a trained psychotherapist so I cannot help you," or "Your problems need much more skill than I am trained to handle." All of the above statements may accurately reflect the helper's belief; however, the parishioner, student or patient has shown a large amount of trust in his minister, teacher, doctor, or counselor by bringing his problems to her. Statements such as the above will undermine the client's trust in his helper's referral judgment and will also make him fearful that his problems are too huge to handle. Instead, the referring helper should affirm the current relationship

and the trust that brought the helper to bring up the subject of his problems. Also, the helper must assure her client that she wants to give him her best assistance in the form of a positive referral linkage with a counselor who has been specifically trained to assist with his type of problem. Further, she must assure her client that she stands ready to maintain her current relationship as minister, teacher, or doctor because that relationship is a valuable one. Finally, the helper should tell her client that if the referral does not work out, he should feel free to return for another referral.

5. *Do not tell the client that he will get over the grief of referral.* If the client feels an attachment for his counselor, then the client may be grieving or clinging to the counselor who is referring him. If the client seems reluctant to move beyond his reaction to the referral, the counselor may become frustrated with the client, wanting him to proceed to the referral resource. The temptation is to point out that this is just one of several relationships and it is time to move on to the referral resource. Further, the counselor may be tempted to reassure the client that once he has met with the new counselor and feels positive about his new counseling relationship, he will get over his feelings about leaving the current relationship.

Clients do not feel consoled by the prospect that they will get over the loss of the current counseling relationship. Counseling relationships are very unique and even if the client does form a positive therapeutic relationship with the next counselor, the new relationship will not replace the former one. Counselors often forget that although they have several clients, the client only has one individual counseling relationship and it is a special one to him.

Case Study: Referral and Client's Grieving

> Karen had been seeing Mary Lou for a year when she found that she was going to move out of state. Karen had to arrange for the referral of several clients. However, Mary Lou seemed to be particularly distressed by Karen's move. Karen had assisted Mary Lou through a major depressive episode, but she was still working on childhood incest issues. When Karen tried to make arrangements to refer Mary Lou to another therapist

highly trained in handling incest issues, Mary Lou resisted. She cried, refused to see the new therapist, and talked about Karen as if she were the only counselor who could help her. Karen became frustrated at Mary Lou's persistent grieving. Finally Karen told Mary Lou that theirs was only one of Mary Lou's many relationships and that she would get over the ending of this relationship as soon as she was connected with her new therapist. Mary Lou was crushed by what she perceived as Karen's callousness. She told Karen that successful therapeutic relationships are not easy to come by and that she resented Karen's blasé attitude. Mary Lou did see another counselor and was able to work through her problems, as well as her feelings of abandonment by Karen. Two years later, Mary Lou wrote Karen a letter explaining her feelings. Mary Lou recalled that when she entered counseling with Karen she felt for the first time in her life that she had someone who understood her and helped her. It was not just counseling, it was the "chemistry" of Karen and Mary Lou together that made Mary Lou work on her problems. Mary Lou confessed that she never got over losing Karen, even though she was able to form a therapeutic relationship with another counselor. Mary Lou observed that what she would have needed was for Karen to stick with her as she grieved, just as Karen had been with her as she tackled her other problems. Mary Lou felt that Karen had thrown their relationship away as relatively insignificant when she told Karen that she would get over the loss of the relationship. although Karen was in some way correct, Mary Lou was not able to hear it at the time of grieving.

6. *Do not say most people feel the same way.* When a client expresses his emotions, apprehensions, and grief over being referred, he is experiencing *his* feelings and not everyone else's who has been referred. Telling a client that his feelings are not unique discounts his feelings. One client said that when his therapist told him that his emotions were not unique, he felt as though he had tried to tell a joke and the counselor person had stopped him in the middle to say that she had heard that one. The feelings experienced at the time of referral are difficult enough for the client to work through without the added burden of deflation at being told his

emotions are not his exclusively. Clients need to be understood, listened to, and accepted. Only when they are afraid that their feelings are crazy or strange is it appropriate to let clients know that their feelings are not unique. Also, there is a difference between telling a client that most people feel the way he feels and telling a client that his feelings are normal.

7. *Do not overexplain or become defensive.* As a client expresses his feelings about being referred, some of his emotions may trigger a defensive reaction in the helper. When this happens, helpers may feel compelled to overexplain their reasons for referral. The helper starts to sound as if she is trying to convince herself that she has made a wise decision or as if she is hiding the real reason for the referral.

Helpers need to be comfortable with other peoples' uncomfortable feelings without becoming defensive or overly talkative. Counselors who become uncomfortable with certain client emotions also tend to try to rescue the client from his own feelings. As clients express their feelings, the counselor or helper must listen, accept, and affirm the client's emotions no matter how defensive or uncomfortable she feels.

8 *Do not dismiss the client.* Of all the mistakes that helpers make during referral, this is the most frequent. The intent of the helper is to leave the responsibility for the referral in the client's hands. However, referral is more than handing a client a list of names and saying good-bye. Referral is a process of transferring the responsibility for therapy to a counselor who is skilled and trained to handle the client's problems. It is similar to the passing of the baton in a relay race.

The referring helper needs to contact the referral resources, work with the client over the issue of being referred, and then, at the proper moment, hand the client over to the referral resource with the knowledge that the client and the referral resource have connected. Handing a client a name or list of referral resources and then wishing the client luck is not referral. At best, it is recommendations. At worse, it is dismissal.

9. *Do not leave clients to their own resources.* Sometimes a counselor will simply terminate a client who still needs and wants

therapy without giving him a list of possible counselors. The client is left to his own resources to make contact with another helper. If a client is still in need or desirous of counseling, the helper has the responsibility to make an appropriate referral.

Case Study: Dismissal

> Dean saw Cally for six months while Cally was suicidal and depressed. Cally was quite resistant to Dean's intervention and he began to lose patience. Cally claimed that Dean did not help her and Dean claimed that Cally did not want help. They decided to terminate. Although Dean knew that Cally still had suicidal ideation, he did not give her a referral. His rationalization was that Cally would not work with anyone. However, Cally still did want help, but she was too depressed and hopeless to make another contact. After several months a counselor-friend of Cally's gave her the name of another counselor. Cally bonded immediately with the new therapist and made remarkable progress.

Dean had made an error in judgment. He believed that since he and Cally had such a stormy relationship, Cally could not work with anyone. Maybe he did not want to believe that someone else could succeed with Cally. There is also a legal issue in this case which will be dealt with in another chapter.

ACCOMPANYING THE CLIENT THROUGH THE REFERRAL PROCESS

Once the decision to refer has been made, the client and counselor talk together about the type of helper the client feels could be of benefit to him. The counselor then tells the client the steps of referral.

1. The counselor will contact the referral resources to ascertain if they are accepting referrals, whether they are interested in

working with a client with a presenting problem such as the client's, and how they wish to receive the referral.

2. The counselor will return to the client with the information that she has obtained. If there is more than one referral resource, then the client can prioritize the names.

3. The counselor gives the client all the names, phone numbers, addresses, and directions for all referral resources.

4. The client makes appointments to see the referral resources or awaits the prospective counselor's call, depending on how the prospective counselor prefers the contact to be made. If the client is very uncomfortable with the referral, the counselor can make the decision to ask the referral resource to join the counselor and client for a session.

5. The client and counselor get together to process the client's meetings with the prospective counselors, to finalize the referral choice, and to say good-bye.

After the process is completed the counselor lets the client know that if he needs any further help with a *referral,* he should feel free to contact her.

Some counselors wait four-to-six weeks and then contact the referral resource and the client to see if the referral has worked well. This is an excellent method of bringing the referral to closure or discovering problems that may have arisen during the referral. See Chapter 8 of this book for follow-up procedure on referrals.

7

Making an Appropriate Client-Referral Match

The decision as to which referral resource to recommend to a client is often limited by the availability of resources in the area. However, assuming that there are several resources from which to choose, the counselor must match the client with the most appropriate prospective counselor. There are five dimensions to be considered in the matching process: skill and training, intellectual style, emotional style, physical situation, and spiritual beliefs.

THE SKILL AND TRAINING DIMENSION

The most obvious match that needs to be considered when making a referral is that between the client's presenting problem and the counselor's skill and training. A counselor who needs to make an appropriate referral must look for referral resources who are thoroughly trained in handling her client's problems. For example, if a women presents herself to a counselor for therapy for depression, the counselor must assess her referral resource list for counselors competent to deal with depression. Since a depressed person may need medication and therapy, the treatment of choice is cognitive counseling coupled with medication, if deemed necessary. The counselor making this referral needs to know her referral resources well so that she can recommend several therapists who use cognitive therapy successfully with clients who are depressed.

Referring a client to another therapist because the therapist is a good friend or needs clients is not a therapeutic referral for the client. This type of referral benefits the counselor and referral resource more than client. An inappropriate referral can lead to the failure of the therapeutic relationship, the client's distrust of the referring counselor's judgment, the client's distrust of the therapeutic process, and therefore, the client's not receiving the help he needs. Further, the mental health profession loses credibility each time a referral is made for any reason other than the client's welfare.

In defense of such actions, counselors sometimes refer to research stating that the most important therapeutic variable is the relationship between counselor and client. Further, they state that since it is difficult to assess whether a therapist and client will "hit it off" they are free to refer as they wish. This attitude arises from a misinterpretation of the research.

Research does support the hypothesis that the relationship is the most important variable in bringing about therapeutic change. However, there is no research that states that this relationship is the exclusive determinant of therapeutic success. In fact, training, skill, and experience are very important variables in developing and maintaining a therapeutic relationship. Further, when a counselor must refer a client, she cannot know for sure whether the client and counselor would be able to engage in a positive counseling relationship. Therefore, the counselor has a responsibility to make an appropriate referral based on the information she does know for certain about the referral resource. The referring counselor's job is to determine that the counselor's abilities match the client's needs.

Case Study: Referral of Convenience

Janet received a phone call from Michelle one day just as Janet was beginning a four-week vacation. Michelle wanted to begin counseling immediately and did not wish to wait a month. Janet, in her haste, referred Michelle to Greg, a counselor who was attempting to increase his client load. Janet had promised Greg all the new clients referred to the agency during her month's vacation. Greg began to see Michelle. Michelle was depressed, suicidal, and anxious. Greg referred Michelle for medication to the psychiatrist on staff, who placed her on appropriate anti-depressant medication. Greg has a master's degree in counseling and was trained and well-respected as a Certified Alcoholism Counselor. He began working with Michelle, uncovering the reasons for her depression. However, Michelle was frustrated. Her depression was not improving, her panic attacks were still a problem, and she still felt suicidal. Greg was also frustrated, because he had never worked with a client who was depressed from something other than alcoholism. His skills in handling depression due to alcoholism were not transferring effectively in Michelle's case. Michelle was becoming scared; her suicidal ideation was increasing. Greg began reading everything he could find on endogenous depression and its treatment. Michelle also tried to read about her depression. Michelle liked Greg and wanted to help him help her. However, Michelle continued to be depressed, suicidal, and anxious. She began to feel even more depressed over the fact that Greg could not help her. Michelle tried to commit suicide using her antidepressant medication. Greg felt guilty because he had hesitated in referring Michelle. He felt that Michelle trusted him and he was fearful of causing her to feel rejected by him.

Greg's skills did not match Michelle's need for counseling. Janet had made the decision to refer Michelle to Greg based on her promise to help increase Greg's caseload. However, Michelle needed a therapist skilled and trained in handling endogenous depression and potential suicide. Michelle's hospitalization helped Greg to see that Michelle needed a differently trained counselor. One was found for Michelle and she began to make progress. The depression began to lift, her panic attacks lessened, her suicidal ideation ceased, and her self-esteem increased. Greg learned a great deal about depression. He also realized his decision to change from an emphasis on alcoholism to general counseling did not automatically result in a transfer of all his skills. Greg arranged for a supervisory relationship to augment his training and enhance his experience.

The case study above illustrates one area of match: skill and training. Actually, the same referral counselor, Janet, had experienced a similar problem when she received a referral of an alcoholic. Janet attempted to work with the young female alcoholic, but the relationship was being manipulated by the client. Janet was not an expert in alcoholism so she was unable to break through the alcoholic's denial mechanism. Janet felt defeated and finally gave up by referring the client to Greg, who was able to use appropriate confrontation intervention.

Generalists pride themselves in their ability to treat a variety of presenting problems. While these counselors do work with many different clients, they must be able to ascertain when a client is in need of a specialist. A counselor should ask herself the following questions in order to assess whether she, as a generalist, should consider referring a client to a specialist:

- Does the client present a problem area which is a recognized specialty, e.g., alcoholism, drug addiction, career development, rehabilitation, child therapy, marriage and family?
- Does the counselor possess the skills necessary to work as a specialist? Or at least, has the counselor received one-to-one supervision on a client who has had this type of presenting problem?
- Has the counselor successfully treated clients with similar presenting problems in the past?
- Is there another more qualified therapist within the client's geographical area who can see the client?
- Can the therapist contract for supervision while working with this client?
- If another specialized individual therapist is not available, is there a group that the client could join to support the current therapy?

If the client is presenting a problem which has traditionally been accepted as a specialty, then the counselor should consider referral if she does not possess the training or experience necessary to qualify as a specialist. At the very least, the counselor should have been supervised by a qualified specialist while working with a previous client with similar presenting problems. By working under supervision, the counselor builds successful treatment plans, and gains appropriate experience in working with clients with special problems. This practice is particularly appropriate to those generalists who work in remote areas where few special resources exist to meet clients' needs. Obviously, a counselor cannot qualify in all specialty areas. Therefore, when a counselor does not have the clinical resources available to refer to a specialist or obtain the special training, supervision is essential while helping a client with a special problem.

In metropolitan areas where there are numerous services and specialists, the counselor should look for a more qualified counselor who does have the skills, training, and experience to help the client with his problem. This does not mean that every client must be referred because there is always a more qualified therapist. The counselor who has adequate experience, skill, and training to deal with a client's problem need not refer unless there are other mitigating circumstances. However, if a counselor has little or no previous experience with the client's problem, then there is reason to consider referral. If the counselor feels she could work with the client provided she had proper supervision, then she can consider this alternative.

It is also helpful for counselors to maintain lists of available support groups which can provide the client with the special information, affirmation, and confrontation targeted to his need.

THE INTELLECTUAL DIMENSION

People process information in several different ways. The intellectual dimension is not based so much on intellectual capability as on the way a person processes information or uses his intellectual abilities. Paying attention to the intellectual dimension in matching a client to a referral resource can reap positive therapeutic referrals. To achieve this, the referring counselor must be aware of the type of intellectual processing profferred by each of her referral resources.

The Inductive Reasoner

An inductive reasoner gathers minutia and then formulates larger generalization based on the smaller pieces of data. People who process information in this manner often have "light bulb" experiences; they benefit from insight therapy, but often appear confused by the myriad of details which they cannot integrate into their generalization. Faced with conflicting data or crises, they tend to retreat into their major life these theses whether they work in the current situation or not. They also attempt to force data into their general systems that do not fit and may become confused and, in some cases, disoriented.

The counselor who works best with the inductive type of intellectual processor is an insight-oriented counselor who is quickly able to sort through details which the client is reporting and find threads of commonality and patterns. The counselor who works least well with this type of processor is one who involves herself with details. Client and counselor then tend to get bogged down in the minutia of each situation without the ability to see the bigger picture.

The Deductive Reasoner

The deductive reasoner tends to have a rigid framework from which he views the world. Important new data are either dismissed if they challenge the established framework or accepted into the framework if they support its structure. Deductive processor tend to split frequently because of their need to make sense of their world at all costs.

The best counselor to work with the deductive type of intellectual processor is one who tolerates a rigid personality style, who can patiently challenge the rigid manner of processing new data, and who can employ cognitive restructuring. The counselor's challenge is to assist the deductive processor, who tends to see things in black and white, to see the greys of life and then eventually to see the colors. The counselor who works least well with these clients is one who tends to be rigid in her own approach to counseling and life. The counselor's rigid nature will tend to collude with the client's to reinforce his rigid thinking and behavior.

The Synthesizer

The synthesizer has the ability both to integrate incoming data into previously established life beliefs and to use it to establish new beliefs. The synthesizer is also able to evaluate his life position and adjust if needed. This type of intellectual processor makes an excellent client. He absorbs new information like a sponge, and can translate the new information into behavior.

These clients work well with most counselors who provide challenge and growth opportunities. However, synthesizers tend to spend most of their processing time in their heads. They struggle with their affective state and may attempt to dismiss their emotional dimension. The intellectual counselor does not work well with these clients. While this counselor stimulates the intellectual process causing the client to improve very quickly at first, the client continues to neglect his affect. The synthesizer needs a counselor who can challenge him to get in touch with, develop, and use his emotional dimension.

The Confused Reasoner

Finally, there is the client who is intellectually confused. These clients are not less intelligent people, but they have never been taught how to process information. They do not know how to distinguish between important and unimportant information. They may spend an inordinate amount of time on the smallest detail and completely dismiss a major issue in their lives. These clients can even appear very dysfunctional because of their inability to order and prioritize their input.

The confused intellectual processor needs a counselor with great patience, who is able to teach him the very elementary processes of decision-making and data-prioritizing. Counselors who move fast with clients, who tend to be very logical and do not understand why others cannot see what they see, and counselors who do not use structure will not work well with these clients. Counselors who work with confused processors must undertake some reparenting of the clients. The counselor must assist the client to learn how to sort through the myriad incoming information, how to prioritize the information, and how to make decisions based on their priorities. This entire process can literally take years.

Case Study: Referral and Intellectual Incompatibility

> James is considered by his colleagues to be a dynamic therapist. His bright, quick mind and gift for insight is envied by many of his friends. James uses cognitive therapy and has a high success rate with his clients. Christine was referred to James through her friend's recommendation. Christine is an intellectually confused processor. Christine had previously been depressed, anxious, and suicidal but currently presented herself as someone who was unhappy and self-defeating. She had trouble making decisions and when she did make a decision, Christine often found that she made the wrong choice based on her poor assessment of information.
>
> At first, James was very confident and positive about working with Christine. He saw her personality disorder as a challenge. However, as the therapy progressed, James began to feel totally frustrated. He knew that Christine was not responding well to him and he was becoming impatient with her. At one point in a therapeutic session, James found himself saying to Christine, "Christine, you must ***think*** about what you

are doing." Christine very honestly responded, "I don't know how." James realized that he did not have the patience to teach her a process that she should have been taught at two-to-four years old. As a synthesizer, James was frustrated with this confused processor. He talked with Christine honestly about her need to learn how to process information. James also affirmed Christine as an intelligent person.

However, James's decision to refer was easy compared to the decision to whom he would refer Christine. James talked to several counselors before he found Robert. Robert utilized primarily an inductive method of reasoning and had worked with other confused processors. Robert was able to work with Christine. He taught her how to prioritize, recognize her needs, sort through her incoming information, and make decisions.

Intellectual Capacity

A counselor who works with very bright clients will frequently avoid the less intelligent client because she feels that the less intelligent client is not as insightful, quick, or prone to progress. This assumption is not accurate. A client's intellectual capacity does not dictate his chances of success in therapy or success with a particular counselor as much as the manner in which he processes information. In fact, a very intelligent person who is out of touch with his emotional dimension may have less of a chance at participating in successful therapy than a person who has average intelligence and who is able to integrate his other dimensions into a holistic appraisal of himself.

THE EMOTIONAL DIMENSION

The emotional dimension of the client is not the diagnosis of the client's dysfunction. Rather, the emotional dimension is the manner in which the client and counselor use their affective state to interact with their environment. Emotional stability, reactions, and defenses should be considered when referring. Since the relationship between counselor and client is so very important to the success of therapy, the careful alignment of counselor and client emotional styles is critical.

Spontaneous Emotional Style

The spontaneous person is an active, engaging person who is an able communicator, expressive and friendly. These clients are enjoyable to communicate with and respond easily to questions and nonverbal behavior. Often they have a quick sense of humor and even when feeling depressed they will still smile and joke through the tears. These clients use denial coupled with humor as active defenses. Spontaneous clients can fool themselves and others, including their therapists, into thinking that all is well with them.

Spontaneous counselors have similar characteristics. They tend to be active counselors, communicating openly and easily. Cognitive therapy, reality therapy, and family therapy are examples of the theories they tend to embrace. They are sometimes overinvested in their client's movement toward health. Spontaneous counselors may need to learn how to use silence and to let the client own his own feelings.

Both spontaneous and reserved counselors can work well with spontaneous clients. A spontaneous client needs someone who will respond to him, but he also needs to slow down his intellectual processing and explore feelings, not just express them. A more reserved counselor will encourage the spontaneous person to stop and feel. The nonexpressive counselor works least well with a spontaneous client. A spontaneous client needs a counselor who interacts with him, responds to his questions, and gives him feedback. A nonexpressive counselor would give the spontaneous client a blank tablet on which to express himself and no direction or feedback.

Nonexpressive Emotional Style

The opposite emotional style from the spontaneous is the nonexpressive style. Nonexpressive clients pride themselves on their "Mr. Spock-like" demeanor. While they may communicate well, their discourse is usually intellectual in nature. Counselors frequently make the mistake of thinking that the nonexpressive client does not feel his emotions. Nonexpressive clients do feel their emotions but they deny the emotive impact and, therefore, do not act or show feelings. They appear cool and confident exhibiting great control. Often they will look with disdain at those who express their emotions freely.

The nonexpressive counselor also experiences her feelings but does not express them to the client. The blank tablet is a purposeful, philosophical statement which allows the client to experience himself by experiencing transference fully. Some therapists mistake the nonexpressive counselor for an unfeeling counselor. This is absolutely not true. Outside the therapeutic milieu the counselor is often a more expressive person.

The reserved counselor who models moderate emotional expression works best with the nonexpressive client. The client will respect the counselor's reserve, and feel safe enough to begin being open to looking at ways to express emotions.

The emotional style least likely to work well with the nonexpressive client is the explosive style. The explosive person differs significantly from the spontaneous person in that she loses control of her emotions, while the spontaneous person expresses her emotions but retains control over them. The explosive style of counseling would not be respected by the nonexpressive client.

Reserved Emotional Style

The reserved style looks at first blush like the nonexpressive style. However, the reserved person does express emotions even though the expression is not as effervescent as that of the spontaneous person. The reserved person experiences his emotions and allows some expression to surface, but then does not allow the feeling to be fully expressed. This type of client stops short of full expression while the nonexpressive person denies his feelings. The reserved client looks like the "cat that swallowed the canary." There is something going on behind the eyes but all of it does not quite make it to the surface.

The reserved counselor carefully monitors her reactions to the client, allowing some emotion to show. The counselor style that works best with a reserved client is either reserved or spontaneous. When working with a reserved client, the most important assets for the counselor to have are the abilities to feel emotions, to explore feelings, and to allow for the identification and expression of all feelings.

The most difficult match for the reserved client is the explosive counselor. The reserved client does tolerate some expression of feeling but does not tolerate lack of control. He would therefore see an explosive personality as unhealthy and out of control. The reserved client also might not enjoy the nonexpressive counselor but might remain in counseling if the nonexpressive counselor matched his intellectual style. Since the reserved client needs to learn about expressing emotions, the nonexpressive counselor may not be the person to aid him in learning this skill.

Explosive Emotional Style

The explosive-style client has no filtering mechanism. All emotions that are felt are expressed, and, at times, are overly expressed. While it is hoped that few counselors would have this emotive demeanor, some counselors may be so spontaneous as to appear close to the explosive style. Clients of this style are overpowering, often demand their own way, and come to counseling because of their inability to get along with people. While the word *explosive* tends to evoke an image of anger, the explosive style can also erupt with laughter, tears, and hugs, or plunge to the depths of despair. Explosive clients are quite histrionic and need plenty of boundaries.

The counselor who works best with the explosive client is one who can provide an atmosphere of structure. The counselor can be reserved, spontaneous, or nonexpressive as long as she can set and maintain limits, confront inappropriate behavior, and avoid being manipulated by the client's outbursts.

An explosive or depressive counselor works poorly with the explosive client. However, since healthy counselors are seldom explosive or depressive as a style of being, the referring counselor can focus on the counselor's ability to handle these overly emotive and manipulative clients.

Depressive Emotional Style

The depressive-style client may or may not exhibit the clinical symptoms of depression that would qualify him for a DSMIII-R diagnosis of depression or dysthymia. The emotionally depressive client has usually begun turning off his emotions in childhood due to trauma or pain until as an adult he is unable to feel. The cost of eliminating the feeling of pain is the elimination of all other positive feelings as well. These clients do not feel sad, depressed, dysphoric, or unhappy. These clients do not feel. Some depressive clients have one emotion left after they have turned all others off. This one emotion is usually anger. The difference between the nonexpressive client and the depressive client is that the nonexpressive client feels emotion and then denies his feelings, while the depressive client does not have feelings he can easily identify. Often the depressive client is not content with not being able to feel. This attitude also differentiates the depressive client from the nonexpressive client.

The depressive client needs a counselor who can act as a role model by experiencing and expressing emotion appropriately. The counselor should also be able to assist the client in unblocking and expressing early-childhood and present feelings. A helper who is spontaneous or reserved can serve this client well if she possess the skill level to unblock critical childhood emotions and then work with the client's powerful feelings as they emerge. Such clients often have horror stories to tell and it takes a skilled therapist to work with the repressed feelings and memories. However, if the client is motivated and open to change, the rewards are worth the hard work.

Case Study: Referral and Emotional Incompatibility

Julie was experiencing a very difficult time in her marriage when she decided to see Scott, a counselor who was very skilled in working with couples. Scott was a nonexpressive person who used cognitive restructuring and family structure techniques to introduce change. Scott worked with Julie, a depressive emotional style client, for several weeks. Julie's husband of twenty years refused help and Julie knew that the end of her marriage was inevitable, but she also knew that ending her marriage was not her major personal problem. Julie had no feelings, and yet she had always been able to accomplish anything that she set her mind to do. Julie approached Scott with her desire to feel, but Scott, in his task-oriented, nonexpressive manner, gave Julie information about how to gain a divorce. Julie explained that she was confused about the divorce because she was confused about herself. She was able to express her anger and her ideas, but nothing more. She asked Scott to assist her in learning to feel and to express her feelings, because she was particularly worried about her lack of maternal feelings for her two daughters. Scott was frustrated with Julie, though he never showed it. He believed that Julie's solution was a divorce, and he though that she would feel better if her husband was not able to harass her.

Julie and Scott were at logger-heads over the differences in their perception of the etiology of Julie's problems. Julie was not moving on the divorce and Scott was unable to identify with Julie's preoccupation with feelings. Scott decided to refer Julie to another therapist. He consulted his supervisor, who recognized Julie's need to be in touch with her feeling dimension. Julie was referred to Kelly, a very spontaneous counselor who was skilled in helping clients get in touch with their feelings. Julie needed the role modeling that Kelly was able to provide. The relationship between Julie and Kelly assisted Julie in exploring her childhood pain and in looking honestly at her current living situation. Julie began to see the painful patterns in her life and began changing them. Through the reawakening of her emotions and emergence of painful memories, Julie was able to look at her marriage as one of her self-defeating patterns. The referral was extremely therapeutic for Julie. She returned to Scott to thank him for recognizing that she needed a different type of counselor.

THE PHYSICAL DIMENSION

The physical dimension can involve many areas such as the client's perception of his own body, the manner in which he treats himself physically, whether he abuses himself, the existence of any debilitating handicaps, his previous health history, his current medical history, the existence of any substance abuse, and current medications. When referring a client, the referring counselor will not necessarily have all of the above information to consider. However, there are several areas that one needs to consider in order to assure that the client and counselor are able to work together.

1. Does the client have any physical disabilities that would necessitate referral to a counselor who is equipped to work with the disability? For example, if the client is unable to climb stairs, the helper needs to be aware of the referral resource's physical layout so that she does not refer the client to a referral resource who does not have handicap access.
2. Does the client have any special transportation problems? The client may need a counselor who is near a bus stop, close to subway access, or within walking distance.
3. Does the client have any physical addictions that need to be considered in the referral? For example, if a client is an alcoholic, then the referral needs to be made to an inpatient clinic where the alcoholism can be brought under control before outpatient therapy can be considered.
4. Is the client currently on medication? A client who is on medication or who is in need of medication would need to be

referred to a psychiatrist or physician for a medication evaluation at the beginning of therapy. This is especially true for clients who are hallucinating or suffering from bipolar or unipolar disorder. The referral can be made directly to a psychiatrist or to a referral resource with the knowledge and resources to network with the medical community for hospitalization and medication.

THE SPIRITUAL DIMENSION

Of all the dimensions that referring helpers can call upon, the spiritual dimension is the least considered by helpers and the most misunderstood. Secular counselors tend to ignore this dimension of their clients' lives. Pastoral counselors and ministers believe that this dimension is one of great importance.

The spiritual dimension refers to the client's belief in a power greater than himself. The dimension includes personal beliefs, values, church-connectedness, and personal philosophy of life. The spiritual dimension is often mistaken for a person's religion, when actually formal religion is only one part of the broader area of spiritual experience. One reason many counselors do not consider the spiritual dimension in their counseling is that religion is a subject, like politics, which many people are taught to avoid. Discussing a person's religious belief may tempt a counselor to become judgmental, especially if the counselor is trying to assist the client to change his values and beliefs.

In addition, many psychologists have theorized that belief in God or participation in religion is a form of pathology. This assertion has not been helped by the many wars started in the name of faith. Nor has it been helped by guilt-inducing methods used by many churches to instill obedience, charity, and a fear of hell.

On the other hand, 66 percent of United States citizens actively participate in church activities (Larson, 1986) and most nonaligned self-help nonchurch groups embrace a power greater than themselves as the only means toward health and abstinence. The question, then, as to where the spiritual dimension belongs in the counselor's office and specifically during the referral process is an important one.

Perhaps the first place to begin assessing the spiritual dimension is to identify the differences between formalized religion and personal faith. A client's personal faith is his own unique set of beliefs, values, and philosophy of life, while formalized religion is the means by which the person chooses to demonstrate his faith. Further, the church with which a person connects may have certain established dogmas, doctrines, tenets, and practices which the individual may personally reject while still belonging to the church.

A counselor may wish to avoid talking about a client's church, but she cannot avoid talking about his beliefs. These impact greatly on the client's perceptions, attitudes, behavior, reactions, and emotions. Suspending judgment is an important part of the counseling relationship which must extend to the spiritual dimension as well. The counselor has to listen, understand, and connect with her client on all dimensions so that the client can examine his life's presuppositions. Like the other dimensions discussed so far, the spiritual dimensions needs attention during the counseling and referral processes. Further, without understanding how a client views life, himself, others, and God, the counselor is working at a disadvantage in knowing and understanding the client and enabling him to change.

In order to ascertain a client's spiritual dimension, the counselor should listen for the client to reveal:

1. What he believes is the purpose of life;
2. What the role he plays in life;
3. Who he considers "others" to be;
4. The belief he has in a supreme being, or the absence of such a belief;
5. How his beliefs influence his everyday life;
6. What values he holds.

If the helper is not a counselor who has been treating the client but is simply acting as a referral agent, then many of the items under the spiritual dimension may be difficult to thoroughly assess.

However, if the client is willing to talk, the referring helper can ask some simple questions that may help.

- Do you believe in a supreme being? If not, what do you believe?
- Would you want your belief to be a part of your counseling? How much a part?

When evaluating the referral resources the questions that may be appropriate are:

- Does the counselor have a belief in a supreme being?
- If a client has a belief system which he wishes to discuss, is the counselor comfortable and qualified to help him address it?

There is no need for counselors to shy away from this dimension. The counselor need not be of the same faith or embrace the same belief system in order to be of help to the client. It is not necessary for the counselor and client to share the same religious faith, any more than they need to share the same sex, race, or background. What is important is that the counselor have an open demeanor, accept differences, and be able to enter the client's inner world.

If a client does have a faith in a supreme being and wishes to talk about the spiritual dimension, then the referring helper needs to respect this wish and refer to a resource who is willing and able to deal with the client's belief system. If a client does not express faith in a supreme being, the client's belief system and value system still need to be a part of the counseling discussion. The important issue is to select a counselor who would not be prone to see the client as more or less healthy depending on whether the client shares her beliefs or not.

The matching of a client and counselor in the spiritual dimension is more a matter of what not to do than what to do.

1. Do not match a deeply religious person with a helper who sees religion as unhealthy.
2. Do not send an atheist or agnostic to a counselor who sees atheism or agnosticism as a pathology.

3. Do not assume that all pastoral counselors or religiously affiliated counselors are out to convert clients.

4. Do not assume that if a counselor or client does not speak about his faith it is not important to him.

5. Do not be afraid to ask a client who is to be referred how important his faith is to him.

Case Study: Referral and Spiritual Incompatibility

> Brian started seeing Rick because of Rick's dissatisfaction with his life. Rick was a deacon in a local church, an accountant, and a homosexual. Rick was struggling with his homosexuality as it pertained to his faith community. While Rick was comfortable with his sexual preference and choice, he was aware that his church taught that homosexuality was a sin. Brian was not a churchgoer and in fact saw most church practices as contrary to mental health. Brian had trouble understanding why Rick would insist on staying in his church when the church was disapproving of his lifestyle. In addition, Brian had some countertransference issues with Rick's religious preference. Brian's way of dealing with his own differences with his church was to leave and renounce religion as unhealthy. Rick's belief would not allow him to leave. Further, Rick was receiving a great deal of affirmation and support from his church friends. Rick terminated his relationship with Brian because he felt that he and Brian were not a therapeutic match. Even though Rick asked Brian for a referral, Brian said that he could not find a counselor who would be able to work with Rick. Rick knew he needed to work on his feelings concerning his faith as well as several other personal issues, but he had felt totally misunderstood by Brian. Several months later another gay friend gave Rick the name of a pastoral counselor. Rick's relationship with this counselor was a very satisfying one.

In the above case study, Rick had originally felt very positive about his relationship with Brian because he felt especially affirmed in his homosexuality by him. However, Brian's incompatibility with Rick's spiritual dimension and church commitment eroded the relationship to the point of premature termination. Also, Brian was unable to make a therapeutic referral for Rick because Brian had not considered or investigated the need to refer a client to a referral resource who was sensitive to the spiritual dimension.

OTHER CONSIDERATIONS WHEN MAKING A REFERRAL

Same-Sex Referrals

Research indicates that referring mental health professionals tend to make same-sex referrals regardless of the sex of the client, the sex of the referring counselor, or the client's presenting problem (Shullman and Betz, 1979). This practice may be seen as effective by counselors because of the belief that a client can be better understood by someone of the same sex. However, as already stated, the client is better served by a counselor with whom the client has the best chance of forming a therapeutic relationship. In some cases, the client may need a counselor of the opposite sex to assure the establishment of trust. For example, a young woman who was sexually abused by a female babysitter and abandoned by her mother might, initially, be more able to trust a male therapist. Nevertheless, some clients request a counselor of a specific sex or may need to consider seeing a counselor of a specific sex to work through some special issues. When a client requests a male or female, the referring helper should try to arrive at a referral resource who meets his need. More and more frequently, homosexual clients are requesting counseling with homosexual counselors or, at least, with counselors who are nonjudgmental in their attitudes toward sexual preference. The referring counselor should be aware of counselors in her area who are compatible with homosexual clients.

Cultural and Racial Issues

There is a plethora of recent journal articles, books, and research on the importance to counselors of studying cross-cultural issues. The client who is of a different culture or race than his counselor may feel uncomfortable at first, while the relationship is developing. This can be avoided if the client can be matched with a counselor of the same race or culture. If this is not possible, then the referring counselor should be keenly aware that the referral resource must be sensitive to and cognizant of cross-cultural issues. The client is the best source of information as to how important having a counselor of the same culture or race is to him.

Geographical Proximity

A client must be able to travel to the therapist's office. This fact may appear to be an obvious consideration; however, it is amazing how many referring helpers are oblivious to this concern. Clients with personal transportation may have the ability to travel longer distances then those who rely on public transportation, but they may still have an outer limit of driving time that they are able or willing to invest in order to reach the therapist's office. The best solution, before giving the client a list of names to call, is to ask the client how far he is willing to travel or what areas are the most convenient for him. Clients may be faced with the choice of two counselors; one perfectly matched to his needs but at a distant location, the other more proximal but not quite as perfect a match to his needs. The choice would then be the client's but he would be more able to make an informed choice.

Financial Resources

Clients usually must consider their financial resources when they make the commitment to counseling. Some clients have insurance that will cover a portion of their fees. Others, however, may not have any insurance coverage for outpatient therapy. Whether a therapist is able to collect third-party payments depends, in great part, on each respective state's laws, the degrees held by the therapist, the type of licensure or certification held by the therapist, and the insurance company's policies. When a client has insurance coverage and a counselor is qualified to receive third-party payment, then the match is favorable to both parties.

However, when a prospective client does not have insurance or when a counselor cannot receive third-party payment, then the client and counselor must negotiate the fee so that it is fair for both therapist and client. Some counselors are willing to negotiate a fee and others are not. The referring counselor should have knowledge of the referral resource's policy regarding fees and her ability to receive third-party payment. Do not overlook the many counselors who work at nonprofit agencies and mental health centers which have sliding fee scales where the client's fee is based on his ability to pay.

CONCLUSION

Matching a client with an appropriate counselor is a major responsibility. The referring helper must learn about the many referral resources available to her and interview the prospective client in order to ascertain the client's needs. Although in many instances the referring helper may not have the time to assess all the various dimensions of both the client and the referral counselor, she should assess as many of the dimensions as possible in order to assure that the referral resource is a therapeutic match.

8

The Referral Follow-up

Once the client has been connected with his new mental health professional, the referring helper still has some final, limited responsibility in the form of the follow-up. There are two basic reasons to follow up on a referral: to assess the referral procedure so that adjustments to the process can be made if necessary, and to assure that the client was able to connect with the new counselor and that a therapeutic relationship has begun. The amount of follow-up will depend to a great extent on the counselor's theoretical and philosophical stance with respect to her relationships with her clients.

Ethically, the responsibility for making an appropriate referral ends when the counselor gives the client a list of referral resources and has made contact with the referral resources to alert them to the possibility of the client's contact. Many helpers allow their responsibility to end with the above completed objectives, not investigating whether or not the client followed through unless they happen to encounter the referral resource later and think to ask. This approach places the primary burden of responsibility for the referral on the client.

Other clinicians feel more responsibility for the referral. They will call the referral resource within a few days to ascertain whether the client followed through with the referral. If the client did not follow through, then the counselor may call the client to assess if the referral process has faltered in some way and to offer to make another referral if necessary. These helpers are invested in the referral process and feel responsible for keeping this procedure from breaking down. These counselors assume the initial responsibility for the referral, and then, once the contact between referral resource and client is made, shift the responsibility to the new counselor and client.

Still other counselors are highly invested in the referral process and not only make the initial contact with the referral resource but also follow up with both the new counselor and the client to ascertain if the referral has worked well for both parties. These helpers assume the primary responsibility for the referral process and the follow-up and then stand ready to assist with another referral if the first is not successful.

The helper who feels that referral follow-up is not necessary embraces a medical model of intervention in which the follow-through responsibility rests with the patient. Further, if the referral resource wishes information from the referring counselor, then it is the referral resource's responsibility to request such information.

The helper who feels that the referral follow-up is important and necessary to the therapeutic process embraces the humanistic model of intervention in which the client's welfare and the referral process are important responsibilities that are shared with the referral resource.

THE IMPORTANCE OF COMMUNICATION

Whichever model the therapist employs, it is important for her to communicate her follow-up preference to others to establish a clear understanding of where the responsibility for the referral follow-up lies. Without this understanding, clients may fall through the cracks of referral.

Case Study: the Referral Follow-up

> Joyce is a psychiatrist who found it necessary to refer Barbara to a mental health professional. Joyce gave Barbara the names of three counselors, believing that she had communicated to Barbara that she should contact one of them for counseling. Barbara thought that Joyce was going to contact one of the therapists on her behalf. Both Joyce and Barbara waited in vain for a telephone call from the new counselor. Two months later, Barbara found a new counselor, Ellen, by herself. Ellen sent Joyce a release of confidential information to obtain copies of Joyce's files on Barbara. Joyce did not understand why Barbara was seeing Ellen because Ellen was not one of three names she had given Barbara. Joyce refused to cooperate with Ellen because she did not know Ellen or her credentials. Joyce called Barbara and insisted that Barbara contact one of the names on her list. Barbara felt confused and betrayed. Barbara recounted to Ellen what had happened with Joyce. Ellen became angry and told Barbara that she would find her a "good" psychiatrist. Barbara wanted professional counseling, but needed her counselor and psychiatrist to work together. Barbara began to feel that the very helpers on whom she relied were no healthier than herself. Barbara dropped out of counseling and ceased seeing her psychiatrist.
>
> Six months later, Barbara was having a very difficult time and decided to try counseling again. This time she connected with her pastor, who made a referral.

The above situation could have been completely avoided. Joyce could have written the referral instructions down for Barbara or had an instruction sheet printed for all her referrals, and then added the names of the referral resources appropriate for Barbara. Joyce invested a great deal of thought in the three referral resources for Barbara and cared deeply that Barbara become connected with a professional counselor who could help address her needs. However, Joyce's medical model did not serve her well because she did not assume responsibility to communicate to Barbara exactly what she desired to have happen.

Ellen, too, could have tried to overcome the communication breakdown by contacting Joyce directly and requesting a meeting. Instead, Ellen felt judged and dismissed by Joyce and reacted with anger, eventually losing the client because of her reaction.

Both helpers wanted to help Barbara but neither was able to be therapeutic with her, and the resulting referral process was non-therapeutic for her as well.

At first glance, it may appear that if Joyce had used a more humanitarian model to approach Barbara's referral, the added communication might have yielded a more positive result. This may or may not be true. If the follow-up communication is unclear, the referral may still not work. For example, even if Joyce had alerted the three referral resources that they might receive a call from Barbara, Joyce would probably never have known if Barbara failed to follow through with the referral since each counselor would assume that one of the other counselors had been contacted. And Barbara would still be awaiting the counselor's phone call. If Joyce had contacted Barbara in four-to-six days to see if she had followed through with the referral, then Joyce would have discovered the confusion in communication. However, if Joyce had waited only two months to follow up, then the same problem would have occurred since Barbara would already have started counseling with Ellen.

To avoid the problem, Joyce needed either to have communicated her medical-model referral process more clearly, or to have adopted a more humanistic model of timely follow-up to prevent the client from falling through the cracks.

Referral Under the Medical Model

A helper wishing to adopt the medical model of referral should communicate to both the client and the referral resources what her referral process entails. She needs to develop a written handout explaining how the referral works and who is expected to do what.

1. The handout should state:
   a. that the client should make the contact with the new helper;
   b. that the client should mention the referring helper's name;
   c. that the new therapist should send a release of confidential information to the referring helper immediately (this contact informs the referring helper that the client has followed through with the referral).
2. The handout should have a place for the names, addresses, and phone numbers of the referral resources and should tell the client how to contact them.
3. Finally, the handout should contain the referring helper's name, address, and phone numbers. See Appendix A for sample forms.

Referral Under the Humanistic Model

A referring helper wishing to employ a more humanistic model of referral must also communicate to everyone involved what is expected of him or her.

1. The referring counselor prepares a handout for the client which contains:
   a. the name, address, and phone numbers of each referral resource;
   b. the referring counselor's name, address, and phone numbers;
   c. instructions as to whether the client should contact the new counselor or the new counselor will contact the client;
   d. instructions that if the referral does not meet his needs, the client is free to contact the referring counselor for additional suggestions.
2. The referring counselor waits no more than two weeks to contact the referral resource to ascertain whether the client has

made an appointment. If the client has followed through, then no other calls need occur.

3. Some referring counselors prefer also to follow up with the client at some point after the referral, to allow the client to express his satisfaction or dissatisfaction with either the referral process or his new counseling relationship. If the referring therapist decides on this action, she should make the follow-up call within two weeks.

WHEN THE REFERRAL DOES NOT WORK

In some instances the therapeutic referral does not culminate in a therapeutic relationship. This can happen when the client does not follow through, when the client does not feel compatible with the referral resource, when the referral resource does not follow through, or when the referral resource makes another referral. Whatever the reason, the referring helper may want to assist the client in finding a new referral resource.

Lack of Client Follow-through

Referring counselors may feel frustrated when clients do agree to referral but do not follow through. This common scenario can lead a referring helper to cease following up on referrals, or worse, to cease investing energy in producing appropriate referrals. However, referring counselors should not allow themselves to succumb to frustration. In some instances their follow-up efforts may spur the client to follow through with the referral after all.

Sometimes clients who do not want to be referred may appear to accept the counselor's list of names and her logic as to why referral is necessary, but then not follow through. A client who is not able to be honest about his feelings regarding referral is likely to continue to mask his real feelings when the counselor calls to follow up on the referral. he may make excuses about why he has not followed through and may even tell the helper that he will contact the new counselor and then not follow through again. Such clients have made up their minds that they will not see anyone who is recommended to them, and the counselor will be unable to convince them otherwise. In this instance, the referring counselor has no alternative but to allow the client the right to choose to remain unhealthy.

Some clients who have not followed through with the referral are ambivalent about being referred. A call from the referring helper expressing concern about the client's lack of follow-through on the referral can often encourage the client to move ahead with the referral, especially if the client is given an opportunity at this time to express any unresolved feelings concerning or questions regarding the referral.

Finally, some clients simply procrastinate about making the contact with their new counselor. They will talk about their busy schedule, a minor crisis, inability to reach the counselor to set an appointment, or lack of funds. The follow-up phone call will usually encourage the client to act. One client said, "Your phone call tells me that you care about my following-through more than I cared about myself." She called and made an appointment with the new counselor the next day.

Client-Counselor Mismatch

A client may not feel compatible with his new counselor after having met with her for a session or two. This client is in a difficult position. Some clients blame themselves for the failure of the new counseling relationship while others blame the new counselor or even the referring helper. For still others, the incompatibility is confusing, causing them to doubt what they feel and how they should express themselves. Some of the symptoms of incompatibility are skipping appointments, being late for appointments, or refusing to discuss certain subjects. Since these symptoms can also indicate resistance, counselors must be cautious about labeling all symptoms that appear to postpone therapeutic intervention as incompatibility. Resistance reflects the client's inability to participate in the very therapeutic activity which can help him to health. However, the client simply may not bond with the new therapist because of lack of trust, feeling he is not being heard, disliking the counselor, or feeling judged by the counselor.

To ascertain whether resistance or incompatibility is causing the symptoms, the counselor can:

1. Ask what counseling the client has had previously and if he felt the therapy was successful. If the client has formed successful therapeutic relationships previously, then the client is probably not bonding with the counselor rather than demonstrating resistance.
2. Determine whether the client works hard while in a given session but misses many sessions. If so, then probably the client is resistant to counseling rather than not compatible with the counselor.
3. Ask the client about the perceived, resistance-like behaviors and watch the client's reaction. If the client talks about needing to take counseling slowly until he feels enough trust to share his innermost feelings, then the counselor should consider that compatibility may be at the center of the resistance-like behaviors. If the client becomes defensive, denies the behaviors, or rationalizes the behaviors, then the counselor should watch for resistance.
4. Mention the possibility of referral to another counselor who is skilled and trained to assist the client with his particular problem. If the client quickly agrees to see someone else, then the client is probably feeling incompatible with the new counselor.

The follow-up phone call to the new counselor may reveal a problem in forming the new therapeutic relationship. The follow-up call will allow the two professionals to explore the problem of compatibility and to discuss whether an additional referral is necessary. This telephone call will also let the new counselor know that she is not alone in the decision to keep or refer the client.

During this time of follow-up, the new counselor may become defensive and deny that there is any difficulty with the new relationship. The referring counselor should support the new counselor's perception and carefully explain that the call is simply a routine follow-up on the referral. If the referral resource suggests that something is not working between herself and the client, then the referring counselor can offer support in reassessing the referral and together they can decide if and how the client should be approached about another referral. If the new counselor appears uncomfortable with or defensive about the idea of a follow-up phone call to herself or the client, then the referring counselor must respect the new counselor's position and not make any personal contact with her or the client. The follow-up phone call could be perceived as interfering with the new counselor's work in establishing the new therapeutic relationship. If this is the case, the referring counselor can send a short follow-up note or postcard to the client and to referral resource in which she states that she is pleased to have made the referral and hopes that the new therapeutic relationship is productive and health-producing for both the client and counselor. She can conclude by stating that if she can be of any further help with the referral, they can feel free to contact her.

Any follow-up contact with the client should always emphasize:

1. Concern for the client's welfare;
2. That the contact is *only* a follow-up;
3. That there will be no further contact unless the client initiates it;
4. That the new counselor and not the referral counselor is the client's therapist.

The follow-up contact with the client should never be:

1. An interference in the therapeutic relationship;
2. A therapeutic session;
3. A excuse to check up on the new therapist's counseling job;
4. An attempt to snoop into the client's therapeutic issues;
5. An attempt to change the client's mind about his new counselor.

If the follow-up reveals an incompatibility between counselor and client, the referring counselor must leave it to the present counselor to make another referral. However, if the client has stopped seeing the new counselor, then the referring counselor can help the client with another referral.

Lack of Follow-through by the Referral Counselor

Referring helpers who follow-up on a referral may find that the client attempted to follow through on the referral but the referral resource failed to return the client's calls. The referral resource may even have made an appointment with the client and then failed to keep it. Clients might not call the referring counselor to inform her of the problem with the referral. The client may even feel bitter and blame the referring counselor for the failure of the referral. The follow-up will reveal the problem and the telephone call or written note can begin a reconciliation process so that the client can gain trust in the next referral.

A Subsequent Referral

The referring counselor may follow up on the referral, only to find that the referral resource referred the client to another helper. The referring counselor may feel betrayed, angry, or frustrated that the time and effort that she invested trying to effect a therapeutic referral was wasted. However, the referring helper must let go of responsibility for the counseling and any subsequent referral, once the referral is made. The follow-up process is only for the purpose of assessing if the original referral process was efficacious and trouble-shooting any problems that may have arisen. The fact that the new counselor made another referral is not a problem. If the referring helper trusts the referral resource enough to refer a client to her, then the helper needs to trust the referral resource enough to accept her decision to refer the client on to another therapist.

THE ROLE OF THE REFERRAL RESOURCE IN THE FOLLOW-UP

The referral resource who accepts the referral of a client has several obligations. The first obligation is to the client. The referral resource needs to contact the client in a timely manner and set up the earliest available appointment. If the referral resource cannot arrange to see the client in a timely fashion, then she should contact the referring helper in case the referring helper wants to contact another referral resource who may be able to see the client sooner.

The referral resource is also obligated to give the referring helper feedback information about the referral process. She should let the referring helper know that she has received the referral and has successfully arranged a session with the client. It is a good business practice for the referral resource to send a thank you note to the referring helper. The referral resource also should let the referring counselor know if the procedure of the referral functioned well for all concerned. It is important that both helpers critique the referral process, in order to make future referrals smooth and error-free.

9

Supervisory Issues in Referral

The goal of supervision is to provide the counselor with another, objective set of eyes on her relationships and working processes with her clients. This supervisory relationship is akin to the counseling relationship; it requires trust, honest feedback, and a genuine alliance which is oriented toward client growth. The major difference between a counseling relationship and a supervisory relationship is that the former focuses on the client and the therapeutic relationship while the latter focuses on the counselor, the client, and the relationship between the two. It is therefore imperative that a supervisor be able to recognize when a counselor should consider referring a client, be aware of how the referral process operates, and know where the community's referral resources are located.

Even though the counselor and supervisor work together effectively to help the counselor be more effective in helping her clients, a counselor may view the need to refer a client as a failure and therefore resist the referral. The supervisor can also become susceptible to the feeling of failure if referral is necessary. A supervisor needs to remind himself that he is not the counselor and has not failed if the counselor must refer a client. In fact, one of the major responsibilities of supervision is to carefully monitor the counselor's readiness to work with clients and recommend referral when necessary. If a supervisor has identified too much with his supervisee, then enmeshment can prompt the supervisor to have to confront many of the same emotions about referral that counselors experience, which are discussed earlier in this book. When enmeshment occurs, the supervisor may not be as available to the counselor to assist with the necessary sorting and processing of the referral decision. To keep the supervisory relationship on a professional plane, the supervisor must view the relationship as he would view a counseling relationship where he is the facilitator, the enabler, the objective cojourneyer, but not the enmeshed alter ego of the client or counselor.

The supervisor must learn about the counselor's abilities, growing edges, goals, personal strengths, emotional vulnerabilities that could lead to countertransference issues, spiritual dimensions, values, physical assets or liabilities, intellectual processes, educational preparedness, and previous supervisory experiences. The counselor in turn will be assessing the client's style of life, assets, liabilities, etc. The supervisor then must look for the parallel processes occurring between client and his environment and the counselor and her environment. In most instances the parallel processes are interesting, enlightening, helpful, and important to the understanding of why the counseling relationship is or is not developing. Looking at the parallel processes will often further the counseling relationship and the counselor's understanding of the client because it helps the counselor understand herself better. However, there are times when the parallel processes are too intense, causing the counselor to be unable to assist the client to change because of her own countertransference issues. The supervisor plays a critical role in the identification of the parallel client-counselor processes and the resulting countertransference issues. Also, the supervisor must often be the first person to raise the issue of referral with the counselor and precipitate the debate about whether or not the client must be referred.

Some counselors resist referring a client even when the countertransference is obviously interfering with the counseling relationship. This counselor may not be objective enough to determine the problem and may be tenacious enough to believe that she can overcome any problem interfering with the client's progress. In such a case supervisors need to stress several issues:

1. The countertransference is apparent and is interfering with the client's therapy.
2. The counselor may be able to work through the countertransference, but while she is effectively working on her issues, the client deserves attention to *his* therapeutic issues.
3. The client's well-being is the prime concern and he deserves a counselor who does not have major countertransference issues with him.
4. Referring the client is the ethical and professional thing to do.

Other counselors want to refer every client with whom they struggle even slightly. Such a counselor has little confidence in herself and doubts her own skills to excess, causing her to believe that every struggle with a client is countertransference. While the counselor will sometimes need to refer, the supervisor's job becomes one of affirming and assuring the counselor that she is capable of handling the troublesome client.

Supervisors will usually be working with counselors who fall in between these two extremes. These counselors have a realistic view of their strengths and growing edges and, as they gather experience, they also gather confidence in handling the more difficult clients. With these counselors, supervision consists of pointing out the counselor's blind spots and assisting the counselor with her professional growth.

To assist a counselor with the issue of whether a client needs to be referred, supervisors can use the following questions:

- Do the client's problems far exceed the counselor's training and ability at this time? If so, then the supervisor should recommend referral to a more skilled therapist.

- Does the counselor's countertransference interfere with the therapeutic process? In order to ascertain if this problem exists, the supervisor should observe the following areas to determine the extent and validity of the interference.
    1. Does the counselor hear the client say things that the client is not saying? For example, is the counselor hearing the client talk about being sexually attracted to her when the client is really talking about feeling emotionally close to her? The supervisor can pick up this misperception by listening to audio tapes or watching video tapes of the sessions.
    2. Does the counselor appear to be pushing the client in one area while the client is dealing with problems in another area?
    3. Does the counselor appear to be overly invested in the client's mental health so that a client's choice of one option over another becomes a major vested interest to the counselor?
    4. Does the counselor tend to talk about her own similar issues rather than the client's issues?
    5. Does the counselor seem to be daydreaming during the supervisory sessions or the counseling sessions?
    6. Does the counselor appear to be expressing emotions about the client, his situation, or his progress which are overly reactive or judgmental?

- Is the counselor overextended with her client load? Counselors tend to take on slightly more clients than they can comfortably deal with in order to allow for no-shoes, vacations, and terminations. However, supervisors should monitor their supervisees' client loads to help them avoid becoming burned out. The number of clients is only one consideration that can contribute to the stress of burnout. The types of clients that the counselor is seeing can also cause stress. For example, a full-time counselor who has several borderline clients may be overstressed even if her number of clients is lower than usual. A supervisor should assist his supervisee in limiting her caseload to a manageable number and in monitoring the composition of the counselor's caseload. The supervisor must also discuss with the counselor the mental and physical energy with which the counselor operates. When the counselor's energy is being drained by her current life issues, crises or personal activities, then the supervisor should aid the counselor in planning her counseling caseload to avoid becoming overstressed to the point of distress. This will necessitate making referrals of the new clients who would either overwork the counselor or drain the counselor's energy. Counselors will often resist this suggestion from the supervisor because of the financial reward of carrying more cases, loyalty to those referring new clients, or worry that there will not be any more new clients for a while. Supervisors need to work with their supervisees to assist them in understanding the limits of their own energy and how the referral process can work for the counselor as well as for the client.

➥ Does the counselor have a specific client who is resistant to the counselor's intervention? When a supervisor is aiding a counselor with a resistant client, it is important for the supervisor to help the counselor determine whether the client is resistant to therapy in general or to this specific counselor. The counselor may have labeled the client resistant, and while this may appear true, the client may be resisting his current counselor because of a lack of trust or a lack of positive match between client and counselor. The supervisor is in an excellent position to help discern which is more likely to be true because of his objectivity and his additional training. In other areas of this book the subject of referring resistant clients is covered. However, in supervision, the supervisor should assess whether:

1. The client has had successful therapeutic relationships previously;
2. The client is expressing the need for a different type of counselor. (this can include a counselor of a different sex, a different race, a different religious orientation, a different emotional makeup, or a different intellectual style);
3. The client is being pushed too quickly to deal with his issues.

If the supervisor can help the counselor discern the difference between a resistant client and a client who is resisting this particular counselor's work, then the counselor can make a therapeutic referral based on the client's need for a different counselor or may retain the resistant client and work on the resistance with the client.

- Does the client need a specialist? The supervisor must keep in mind that clients may need a specialist and the supervisee may not have the necessary credentials to work with the client. When this occurs, the counselor may resist referring the client because of the bonding that has already taken place. The counselor may being reading about the client's problem and asking for additional supervision so that she is able to keep working with the client. If the supervisor has the special skills needed by the client, then it may be possible for the counselor to continue working with the client if she receives additional supervision on the client's problem. However, the supervisor must take a realistic appraisal of his own skill level and his ability to pass on the information and skills on through the supervisory process. If the supervisor determines that the specialized skills must be acquired through formal education or programmed study rather than supervision, then he must recommend that the counselor refer the client to a specialist. If the supervisor concludes that the counselor can work with the client if the counselor were to receive special tutoring, then the counselor and client can both benefit from nonreferral.

- Do the counselor and client have a positive therapeutic relationship? Assessing a positive relationship between client and counselor is difficult and the supervisor will often have to rely on the counselor's and/or client's self-reports as to whether the relationship is progressing or not. The counselor may be so involved with trying her best to bond with the client that she does not perceive that the client and she are not a therapeutic match. The supervisor can objectively view or listen to tapes in order to assess whether the counselor-client relationship contains trust, positive regard, honesty, genuineness, and caring. Also the supervisor can assess whether the client is sharing his story and beginning to do the therapeutic work necessary to change.

Many counselors rush the therapeutic relationship; in this case, the supervisor must talk with the counselor about taking time in therapy to bond with the client. When a counselor is hasty in trying to establish the relationship in an effort to help the client to change, she may assume prematurely that the relationship already exists. Before any therapeutic work can occur, the relationship must be solidly formed. When this does not happen, the supervisor should ask whether the counselor and client are appropriately matched. The supervisor can assess the emotional, intellectual, spiritual, and physical matchings discussed in other chapters of this book. When a match does not seem to have occurred, the supervisor has the responsibility to bring the issue to the counselor for discussion and possible referral.

Because the lack of a therapeutic match is often a covert rather than an overt issue, the counselor may need time to determine whether or not a referral is appropriate. The supervisor must have patience and perseverance in this area. Above all, the supervisor must not shy away from the discussion about the mismatch.

CONCLUSION

Supervision is a critical part of the entire helping process. When referral is necessary, supervision is invaluable. Not only will the supervisor be an excellent resource for referral possibilities, but also the supervision provides an opportunity for the counselor to process the decision and the reasons for referral.

10

Professional, Ethical, and Legal Concerns

The decade of the 1980s heralded a new awareness of the helping professions' liability to the potential legal ramifications of professional relationships with clients. All helpers need to be keenly aware of their responsibility, professional identity, limits to confidentiality, professional conduct, ethical standards, and vulnerability. While the referral of a client to another helper appears at first glance to be somewhat removed from the more common reasons why helpers are sued, the fact is that referral includes many areas which have been proven in the courts to be the professional's responsibility. While no actual case involving referral has been cited in the literature, the experts do draw on similar actions in other related professions in order to offer helpers guidelines for their actions (Hopkins and Anderson, 1985). Therefore, in the absence of any actual court case that may set a precedent, the courts usually turn to the self-imposed standard of the profession to determine liability and the standard of care that helpers in similar situations would normally be expected to give (Hopkins and Anderson, 1985). Helpers are well advised to act within the guidelines of their respective professions' ethical standards and to readily seek the advice of an attorney who is cognizant of the field's many challenging complexities.

CONFIDENTIALITY

The freedom to exchange ideas and information during referral is absolutely essential to the successful process of a therapeutic referral. However, during the exchange, the client's confidentiality must be a prime concern of the referring therapist. The incompatibility of these two needs can frustrate the very process of referral which is meant to help the client.

According to Hopkins and Anderson (1985), "Confidentiality is the exchange of information between two people in a professional-client situation, in which the confidential relationship has been expressly recognized by statute or by common law." The difficulty arises because each state regulates and defines the term *confidentiality* and further defines who has the right to confidential communications. For example, only two-thirds of American jurisdictions sanction the priest-penitent relationship. Some states extend the privilege to accountants and their clients but do not accord the same privilege to counselors and their clients. Helpers should be well-versed in the statues of their own state of practice. Legally, confidentiality refers to the courts' ability to insist on the counselor's testimony about her client. Most information that is discussed in a counseling relationship will never be of interest to the court of law.

However, the term *confidentiality* also applies in the helping professions to the divulging of information to a third party who has no need or right to receive it. This type of breach of confidentiality is termed by civil courts as the invasion of privacy. It is within this realm that referral can lead to civil action if the client's privileged communication is not protected. When a referral is being considered, the referring helper may feel compelled to speak directly to the referral resources about the client, including the presenting problem, the diagnosis, the reason for referral, and the progress that the client has made thus far. In order to speak to the referral resources without unduly risking a law suit based on the invasion of privacy, the referring counselor can do the following:

1. Have the client sign a release of confidential information permitting the counselor to talk with other professionals who are possible referral resources (see Appendix A for a sample form).
2. When speaking with the potential referral resources, avoid using the client's name or giving any identifying information until the decision is made as to whom the client is being referred. Then the new counselor can receive the necessary identifiers along with the signed release of confidential information.
3. Avoid unfairly injuring the client's reputation with the referral resources. Even if the statements are true, the client may still be injured if derogatory information is communicated to a third party who has no need of the information at the time. Therefore, when contacting several counselors to ascertain which is the best match for the client, it is important to give the pertinent general facts without giving too much information, especially derogatory data, about the client.
4. Make sure that all information that is transmitted both in writing and orally is accurate.
5. Communicate only information that is required for the purpose of referral.
6. Transmit information properly, with the release-of-confidential-information form, by appropriate means and to the appropriate parties. For example, the referring counselor should talk with or write to the referral resource directly, and not give referral information to a secretary, spouse, or colleague. After the referral has been made and the client is seeing the new counselor, she may wish to have copies of the referring counselor's case information. The information to be transmitted must meet all of the above criteria. For example, the client information must be accurate, nonderogatory, limited to the purpose of informing the counselor about the client's previous counseling, and directed only to the new counselor. In addition, the referring counselor should request a copy of the new therapist's form signed by the client

releasing the confidential information. When the information about the previous counseling process is requested, the referring counselor should still make decisions as to what information to include. Factual, objective information on intake forms, tests, or assessments may be transmitted. However, personal case notes of the therapist should not be given to the new counselor. Although it is more time-consuming, both the therapist and the client would be better served if the therapist were to send a case summary, in which she has sorted through all of her impressions, tape recordings, correspondence, goals, ideas, etc., and arrived at a two or three-page synopsis of accurate, pertinent, helpful information presented in a professional manner.

The American Association for Counseling and Development states in its Ethical Standards that

> Records of the counseling relationship, including interview notes, test data, correspondence, tape records and other documents, are to be considered professional information for use in counseling and they should not be considered a part of the records of the institution or agency in which the counselor is employed unless specified by state statute or regulation. Revelation to others of counseling material must occur only upon the expressed consent of the client. (AACD Ethical Standards, 1988)

The above excerpt points out that counselors do not have to routinely transmit all of their collected data on a client simply because it is requested. The counselor accurately summarizes the information *necessary* to the understanding of the client and his therapeutic concerns and this summary becomes the termination synopsis or the referral synopsis which becomes a part of the permanent client file.

One final note of concern about the above excerpt is that although the standard calls for "expressed consent of the client" in transmitting information, the counselor must always think in terms of "expressed *written* consent of the client."

Case Study: Referral and Confidentiality

Aaron and Carl had had a personal and professional relationship for several years. They admired and trusted each other's work and frequently used each other as consultants and referral resources. Aaron had interviewed Kathy twice before he realized that Kathy needed immediate long-term help. Aaron was leaving on vacation and believed that Kathy could not go without counseling for three weeks, so he referred Kathy to his friend Carl. Aaron considered no other counselors for Kathy and told Kathy to go see Carl immediately. Since Aaron was leaving town, he dropped Carl a note intended to fill him in on Kathy. He told Carl not only that Kathy was crazy and manipulative but that he suspected that she was a classic borderline who was trying to seduce him. Aaron warned Carl that this was a difficult case but that he was sure Carl could handle Kathy. Before Aaron left, he called Carl to be sure that he had received the letter and talked with Carl's wife. Because Aaron knew Carl's wife well, Aaron explained why he was calling, mentioned Kathy's name and diagnosis, and once again referred to her as "pretty crazy."

Kathy had not even seen Carl yet and already she was beginning therapeutic work under a cloud. First, Aaron shared information with a third party (Carl's wife) who had no reason to have such sensitive information. Second, Aaron shared his clinical impressions with Carl about Kathy in a derogatory manner and made these impressions known in writing to Carl and verbally to Carl's wife. Finally, Aaron did not consider who could best work with Kathy, engage her in the decision, and then complete the referral. If Kathy ever found out about the letter that Aaron wrote to Carl, the phone call to Carl's wife, and the lack of professional processing of the referral, Kathy could press a civil suit against Aaron for both libel and slander (defamation of character) as well as invasion of privacy. Even if Aaron had Kathy's well-being in mind and acted in good faith, he did not limit his comments to the purpose of referral, he did not transmit the information properly, and he did not transmit the information to only the proper party.

Although Kathy never did find out about the errors that Aaron made, Aaron took undue risk with his actions. While it is true that most clients do not discover the errors that their counselors make, counselors who continually make the same errors of judgment in their referral practices are walking a tight rope of being discovered.

MALPRACTICE AND REFERRAL

While there is no clear guideline as to what constitutes malpractice in a counselor-client relationship, "profession malpractice is generally judged by whether a reasonably prudent counselor in the same or similar circumstance would have acted in the same manner as the counselor" (Hopkins and Anderson, 1985). Obviously, one of the major concerns that arises out of such a definition is whose standard is to be applied to judge whether a counselor was negligent in performing her duty to her client. Because there have been so few cases that can aid in the establishment of "the standard," the courts draw upon similar professions and current professional organizations' ethical standards to measure the helper's performance.

In the area of therapeutic referral, the counselor has a responsibility to continually assess the client's progress and determine whether her intervention with the client is contributing to his progress. The counselor's duty to refer, if the client needs a more experienced therapist, a specialist, or a differently trained therapist, is mandatory. The counselor who refuses or hesitates to refer a client who needs more advanced professional attention than she can offer, could open herself up to action for malpractice because she is obligated to send the client to a competent professional.

The American Association for Counseling and Development states in its Ethical Standards:

> If the member determines an inability to be of professional assistance to the client, the member must either avoid initiating the counseling relationship or immediately terminate that relationship. In either event, the member must suggest appro-

> priate alternatives. (The member must be knowledgeable about referral resources so that a satisfactory referral can be initiated.) In the event the client declines the suggested referral, the member is not obligated to continue the relationship. (AACD Ethical Standards, 1988)

The above excerpt is general in nature as it refers to the "inability to be of professional assistance." These words can mean that the counselor lacks the proper training, lacks the adequate experience, lacks the necessary knowledge, or has countertransference issues with the client.

It is important to note that AACD recognizes the need for a helper to know her environment and community well, so that a satisfactory referral is possible. While no court action has ever been brought concerning referral, the possibility exists that a referring counselor could be held accountable by the courts if she were to refer a client to another counselor knowing full well that the new counselor does not hold the necessary training, expertise, or credentials to deal with the client's presenting problems. Further, the counselor could be held responsible if she does not possess the required skills or expertise to work with a client and does not refer the client to another therapist who does possess the appropriate credentials. This could also be true if the counselor bases her referral on anything other than competence. For example, if a counselor refers the client to another professional because that professional is a friend or is in need of clients, then the referring counselor could be held culpable.

The American Association for Counseling and Development also takes a stand on referral based on a client's ability to pay. In Section A 5 of the Ethical Standards, AACD states:

> In the event that the established fee structure is inappropriate for a client, assistance must be provided in finding comparable service of acceptable cost. (AACD Ethical Standards, 1988)

This statement further iterates that the counselor must know her community resources well, including the various agencies and private practitioners' fee scales and exceptions to the fee scales.

Finally, referral must take place when the counselor has other relationships with the client or prospective client. All professional helping organizations have a statement in their ethical standards forbidding counselors to hold dual roles with their clients except under extreme circumstances. These extreme circumstances are usually limited to the situation where an alternative is unavailable and the person needs counseling intervention. Dual relationships might impair the counselor's objectivity and judgment and thereby interfere with the therapeutic relationship. When dual relationships occur, the counselor must terminate by referring the client to another competent professional. The counselor who does not terminate dual relationships is unduly risking legal repercussions as well as ethical censure.

CONCLUSION

Referral is a critical activity that assists clients in connecting with the most appropriate helper available. The activity needs to be handled with the same sensitivity, concern for the client, and timing that is necessary for a counseling relationship. Therefore, referring counselors need to see the act of referral as a major ethical responsibility that could have legal consequences.

11

Decreasing the Probability of the No-Show Referral

Clients who do not show up for their first appointment following a referral are a chronic problem for counselors. Zinos and Hopkins (1981) found that between 20 and 50 percent of clients do not keep their first appointments while Gould, Paulson, and Daniels-Epps (1970) estimated that a stable 20 to 30 percent of first session clients fail to meet with counselors.

Several investigators have researched the relationships between no-shows and a number of variables, including type of presenting problem, socioeconomic level, education, referral source, clarity of presenting issue, previous counseling/no previous counseling, race, age, sex, and being placed on a waiting list.

TYPE OF PRESENTING PROBLEM AND NO-SHOW ACTIVITY

Clients present themselves for counseling with myriad problems. Certain problem areas tend to yield no-show activity. For example,

Raynes and Warren (1971) found that clients who were referred to a counselor for the purpose of working through loss or grief were less likely to show up for the first appointment than those who were presenting other problems for counseling. Raynes and Warren (1971) speculated, based on follow-up contact with those who did not show, that loss and grief yields overwhelming, immediate reactions that tend to decrease over time. If a client makes an appointment while overwhelmed with emotion but then must wait several days for the first appointment, the most intense feelings of being overwhelmed probably have subsided by the time the appointment hour approaches, so he feels less need for assistance.

One resolution to the no-show client who is presenting a grief reaction is to treat that client as if he is in a crisis and see him immediately rather than waiting for the most convenient time or placing him on a waiting list. If this action is not possible, then a referral may be in order so that the client can be seen while his need is the greatest.

Perhaps mental health professionals tend to assure that if grief normally resolves itself over time, then the client may not need to be seen at all and postponing the appointment allows the client to use his routine coping mechanisms and thereby work through the grief reaction or uncomplicated bereavement on his own. However, another view of this issue is needed. If a client calls for help during his grief, then probably his normal coping mechanisms have not served him well and by entering counseling at that moment, he will learn other means by which he can begin coping with his grief. Learning new skills or having someone with whom he can share his pain who is not engaged in the same grieving process can be very beneficial and growth-producing for the client. If he is not given the opportunity for counseling, then he is not able to grow beyond his current coping style and may also suffer a more complicated bereavement experience later in his life.

Earlier in the book, the subject of how to connect the most appropriate helper with the client was covered. In the case of bereavement, this issue can be extremely important. Bereavement calls for empathy, warmth, and an understanding on the part of the counselor of the intense pain that one experiences when loss occurs.

When referring a client who is experiencing grief, it is imperative that the counselor be available, compassionate, empathic, and caring. Clients who experience the loss of a child, spouse, or parent evoke sympathy in most people and will probably have enough sympathetic ears around during grief. What the client needs is someone who is not experiencing his current loss but is able to empathize with the pain of the loss and then gently help move him toward the resolution of the crisis so that he is at least functioning at the precrisis level of activity with some new skills of his own.

Counselors who take the view of grieving as "Let's get on with life" may not be the best referral resource for the bereft client. This is especially true in cases where the counselor has little empathy for the type of loss that the client is experiencing. For example, a client who is grieving the loss of his beloved pet of fifteen years needs a counselor who understands and is empathic toward the issue of pet loss. For many counselors, animals are not a central part of their lives; they may not even own or enjoy pets. Other counselors are allergic to animals and have never experienced the joy (and pain) of owning a loyal pet. However, for a great many people, pets are a great source of friendship and love. Losing a pet can have a profound effect on the client that is misunderstood or not appreciated. A counselor who is not able to understand this client's grief may recommend a "replacement." To a bereaved pet owner such a suggestion is as repulsive and premature as the suggestion that he can have other children would be to a client who has just lost a child.

Another presenting problem that seems resistant to referral is what clients often call "having a nervous breakdown." Again, Raynes and Warren (1971) found a high correlation between clients who claim to be having a nervous breakdown and no-show activity. While Warren and Raynes do not speculate why this type of client frequently does not follow through with referral, the answer may lie in several areas. Clients who claim that they are having a nervous breakdown may be experiencing an episode of histrionic behavior which often subsides rapidly. Because of the labile nature of histrionic clients, it is not surprising that they would make an appointment when they felt the critical need and then decide against going or forget to go once they no longer were histrionic. Another possibility is that these clients may feel the need to be seen right away and, therefore, find other counselors who are available. Finally, clients who perceive themselves as having a nervous breakdown may tend to hospitalize themselves more frequently than other clients.

To avert the possibility of a no-show, the referring counselor is well advised to determine whether the client needs hospitalization, crisis-management counseling or traditional outpatient counseling. Identifying and defining the problem clearly and succinctly will give the referring counselor an opportunity to hospitalize or refer to an appropriate counselor. If the client appears to be histrionic, then the referring professional could advise the client that his symptoms will probably feel less intense by the time of the first appointment, but that it is still vitally important for him to keep the appointment no matter how much better he feels. By thus directly addressing the labile emotional response of the client, the referring counselor sets the stage for follow-through.

The client who is truly disintegrating needs more than a referral to another counselor. This client may need hospitalization in order to stabilize his reactions. Often this client needs medication and the physical restrictions of a hospital setting. Referring this client to another outpatient counselor sets the stage for a no-show.

A client experiencing a nervous breakdown may also be totally overwhelmed by his current life situation or have lost the ability to cope with situations which he was once able to handle. This client probably does not need hospitalization, but does need immediate care. Therefore, the referring counselor must consider the availability of the new counselor, for this client must not be placed on a waiting list or otherwise postponed.

Deciding which type of nervous breakdown the client is having calls for accurate diagnosis and assessment, which is beyond the scope of this book. The counselor should have highly developed diagnostic skills and seek supervision and/or consultation in order to assist the client in the most appropriate manner. In addition, the following chart may help to sort through the histrionics in order to decide what type of referral is necessary: referral to traditional outpatient resources, hospitalization, or crisis management. Using the statement on the left, the counselor is able to assess the client's state of anxiety. However, because diagnosis is such an intricate process, often more information is needed before a concrete diagnosis can be made; the chart on page 163 is instead only as a guide.

SOCIOECONOMIC LEVEL, OCCUPATION, EDUCATION, AND NO-SHOW ACTIVITY

Gould et al. (1970) found no correlation between clients not showing up for an appointment after a referral and socioeconomic levels, occupation, or education. While many counselors may disagree with the outcome of Gould's research, the fact is that research does not support a relationship between the above variables. However, the dearth of research on referral activities makes drawing conclusions more difficult. Many more studies are needed before clear patterns will become discernable.

REFERRAL SOURCES AND NO-SHOW ACTIVITY

Research results conflict over whether there is a correlation between type of referral source and a client's showing up for the first appointment. Raynes and Warren (1971) found no significant relationship between show/no show and the source of referral. However, Gould et al. (1970) found a positive correlation between type of referral source and show/no-show outcome. According to Gould et al., a positive relationship exists between what they call a convincing referral source and show activity. The convincing referral sources identified by Gould et al. were doctors, lawyers, and spouses. They contend that the more medical, legal, or significant the relationship, the greater the chance of the client's showing up for the appointment. It appears that the referral source must be perceived as powerful, knowledgeable, and influential for the client

ASSESSING THE CLIENT'S REFERRAL NEED IF CLIENT REPORTS HAVING A "NERVOUS BREAKDOWN"

	CLUSTER 'B' PERSONALITY DISORDER: PROBABLY NEEDS TRADITIONAL THERAPY	NEEDS HOSPITALIZATION	CRISIS: NEEDS OUTPATIENT IMMEDIATELY WITH POSS. OF ASSESSMENT FOR MEDICATION
Histrionics are a routine part of client's reactions.	pY	M	pN
The client seems manipulative.	pY	pN	pN
The client is threatening suicide.	M	Y	N
The client is endangering the safety of self or others.	pY	Y	N
The client is attempting to bring attention to himself.	pY	N	N
The client has difficulty following through with therapy or suggestions.	pY	N	N
The client seems to lose touch with reality.	M	Y	N
The client is emotionally available for counseling.	M	pN	pY
The client is expressing that this is the first (or one of only a few) time(s) that he has felt out of control.	pN	pN	Y
The client appears baffled by why this is happening to him.	pN	pN	Y
The client blames others totally for the way he is feeling.	pY	pN	pN
The client appears motivated and interested in exploring self.	pN	pN	pY

Yes (Y), No (N), Maybe (M) Probably Yes (pY), Probably No (pN) to feel positive enough about the referral to follow through with the appointment.

Perhaps the different outcomes of the two studies can be explained by the two different approaches used in the studies. In the Raynes and Warren (1971) study, researchers looked only at the type of referral source, while Gould et al. (1970) researched both the type of referral source and the ability of the referral source to be convincing. Therefore, it would seem that in making referrals, counselors must see and present themselves as professionals so that they are credible to the client whom they are referring.

CLARITY OF PRESENTING ISSUES AND NO-SHOW ACTIVITY

Gould et al. (1970) found that those clients who have the most clearly defined reasons for seeking help tend to show up for the first appointment following referral, while those with the vaguest reasons tend not to show. The referring counselor can assist the referral process by helping the client to define his need for counseling and to understand the need for him to be active and motivated to change. Taking the time to assist the client in formulating his direction in entering counseling will reap a positive referral process and a successful outcome in therapy.

Helping the client to clarify reasons for counseling involves discussing definition, responsibility, and expectations. The definition of a client's need for entering therapy needs to be as concrete as possible. A client who simply states that he is unhappy has not completed the definition process. The referring counselor can ask the client to identify what thoughts, feelings, physical issues, religious beliefs or values, and relationships are contributing to the client's unhappiness. Narrowing the contributors to unhappiness allows the client to begin formulating the direction for his therapy and may actually give the client reason to enter counseling.

The referring counselor can also assist the client to recognize his responsibility for his own health and for the relationships in which he is involved. While the in-depth work is done in the therapeutic relationship, the referring counselor can aid the process by helping the client understand that entering counseling is a positive, growth-oriented activity. The referring counselor can also talk with the client about his responsibility to the counseling process. In this way, the client has an idea about what commitment he is making to therapy.

The final area of discussion can center around the client's expectations of what happens in counseling. Some clients believe that a magical solution will be performed by the counselor. As such a client begins counseling, he will become disappointed with the counselor's participation. However, if expectations for the counseling process are discussed during referral, then the client has a realistic sense of what to expect from counseling and what not to expect. This discussion can increase the probability that a referral will be successful.

PREVIOUS COUNSELING/NO PREVIOUS COUNSELING AND NO-SHOW ACTIVITY

For clients who have already been in counseling and who, therefore, have an idea of what to expect from the process, the referring counselor can determine if the previous counseling was viewed as successful by the client, and further, what he did and did not achieve in his previous relationship. Gould et al. (1970) found that clients who had been in treatment previously had a tendency to not show up for the new referral appointment. Perhaps clients who have had less than successful experiences in the past are reluctant to engage in counseling again. That is why discussion of expectations is so very critical. A client who expects the counselor to fix everything is likely to be disappointed with therapy. He may sabotage the referral by not allowing the new therapeutic relationship to succeed or by not showing up for his appointment. Clients who have had an excellent experience with counseling could also be reticent about trying a new therapist. They may fear that the new relationship will disappoint them because their expectations are so high. The referring counselor can assist both of these clients through a discussion about what to expect from counseling and how each counselor brings her unique style, experience, and expertise to the counseling relationship.

Clarifying Client Expectations

Whether a client has had previous counseling or not, helping him to address his expectations brings the purpose of counseling into focus and leads to more realistic expectations. The following observations about the counseling process can be used as a basis for discussion:

1. Counseling is based on a relationship between counselor and client.
2. The counselor does not have all the answers, however the counselor does have training and experience in normal human development, problem solving, psychopathology, forming a relationship, analyzing interaction, seeing patterns of behavior, and utilization of techniques for improving the human condition.
3. The counseling relationship is built on trust and honesty. If the client is unable to be honest and trustworthy, then the therapeutic experience will not be successful. The counselor must also be honest and trustworthy or the client will not be free to explore important issues.
4. The counselor will attempt to be genuine, nonjudgmental, and supportive of the client. However, the client needs to understand that the counselor must also point out to the client any discrepancies in his behavior/thoughts/feelings and when the client is being self-defeating or self-destructive.
5. While the counseling milieu is one of acceptance and caring, the counselor will need to set boundaries within which the counseling can take place. One young woman had been to four different therapists because she could not find a counselor who "cared." When facing a fifth referral, the referring helper finally asked the

young woman what behavior she considered indicative of being caring. The young woman replied that she wanted her counselor to call or write to her between sessions. The referring counselor took this opportunity to explain the expectations and boundaries of counseling. The fifth referral was successful.

6. The counselor devotes an hour or two (or any specified time) each week solely to the client and his problem. In return the client pays the counselor for her time and expertise.

7. The responsibility for the solution of the client's problem or for the improved health of the client rests squarely on his shoulders. The client spends one hour each week (or any specified time) in the counseling session and 167 hours away from the counseling relationship. How the client utilizes the time away from the counselor is many times more important than time in the counselor's office, first by shear numbers and secondly because of the necessity of transferring the learning and insight obtained in the counseling office to real-life situations.

8. The counseling relationship is a confidential one, but there are limits to confidentiality set by law. For example, a counselor must report any suspected child abuse to the respective state authorities. A counselor must also warn others if the client is threatening to harm them or is threatening suicide or self-harm.

9. The counselor and client must see each other on a regular basis, usually weekly is a minimum, in order for the relationship to form, for consistency of tracking behavior/thoughts/emotions to occur, and for the hour to be utilized to its fullest potential. Change does not happen by just catching up on the client's time away from the counselor.

10. The client and counselor will seek together to define the client's problem and the means by which to arrive at a healthy solution. However, change, even positive change, can affect other relationships negatively. Clients should be aware that sometimes one person in a system will begin to be healthier and in doing so will upset the system. Divorce, loss of relationship, or alienation can occur. On a positive note, sometimes a client's improved mental health can result in closer, more intimate relationships.

11. If the counseling required or requested is for marriage or

family, then the focus of the counseling will be on the relationship not on a specific person. A client who wishes family counseling in order to solve the problem of the acting-out child must understand that the focus will be on the entire family, not on the perceived "problem" child.

12. Counselors are human beings, not superhuman beings, and as such, they find from time to time that they must refer clients because they, as counselors, are unable to be therapeutic with certain clients. Clients need to understand that this referral has little to do with them personally and is in their best interest.

Assisting clients with clarifying their expectations of counseling and their problems will greatly improve the chances of a successful referral. The referring counselor usually does not perceive her role as being as active as the picture presented above. However, one of the major problems with unsuccessful referrals is that the counselor making the referral is sloughing off the client rather than actively and therapeutically connecting the client with another helper. In fact, Raynes and Warren (1971) found that improved referral techniques yielded an increase in referral show rates. Their research supported the hypothesis that referring counselors who listen more fully during referral and who aid in alleviating clients' fears of therapy improved the referral show rates.

RACE, AGE, SEX, AND NO-SHOW ACTIVITY

Raynes and Warren (1971) researched the relationship of race, age, and sex to no-show activity. Their findings supported what many counselors have experienced: that blacks, males, and those under forty years of age are less likely to show up for first appointments. Why these patterns have developed is not clear. Perhaps there is less trust in authority or systems of help in young black men. As suggested earlier, the solution may be to spend a little more time with those under forty, blacks, and males helping to define and clarify expectations of counseling so that they feel more secure in the knowledge of what commitment to counseling means for them and what type of relationship to expect.

WAIT LISTS AND NO-SHOW ACTIVITY

Human services professionals have long used waiting lists when the practice is full and yet clients are interested in seeing a particular person. While Gould et al. (1970) showed no correlation between no-show/show activity and the time between initial call and appointment, they were not explicitly researching wait-listing. Raynes and Warren (1971), however, did specifically include the waiting list variable in their research and found that the elimination of the waiting list increased show rates. It therefore appears that if the client receives an appointment, even if it is a week or two in the future, he will be more likely to follow through with the appointment than if he is placed on a waiting list. One reason for this may be that many wait-listed clients seek alternative help instead of waiting.

WHAT THE REFERRAL RESOURCE CAN DO TO DECREASE NO-SHOW ACTIVITY

So far, the discussion has revolved around what the referring counselor can do to increase show behavior following referral. To further reduce the probability of a no-show the professional receiving the referral can telephone the prospective client to assuage his fear, mail a reminder about the appointment time and location, and decrease waiting time between the initial contact and the first appointment (Zinos and Hopkins, 1981).

Another question to be addressed is what a counselor should do if a client does not show up. While this subject was covered more thoroughly in a previous chapter, the researchers cited throughout this chapter support the follow-up phone call as the single most efficacious way to stimulate the no-show client to reconsider his decision not to enter counseling. The follow-up phone call has stimulated many people to come into a clinic and they have been quite grateful to have been remembered and contacted—as if they were truly lost (Gould et al., 1970).

12

The School Counselor and the Referral Process

School counselors are faced with ever-increasing workloads. While in some schools, school counselors are blessed with student/counselor ratios as low as 350/1, most school districts have much higher ratios, even reaching as high as 1000/1. Even though the American School Counselor Association recommends much lower ratios, the reality is that high student-counselor ratios make it difficult for school counselors to provide services and more likely for them to make referrals to family therapists and other mental health professionals. In addition, school counselors report that more and more school-age children are experiencing emotional difficulties that require psychotherapy (Bobele and Conran, 1988).

Despite the increasing ratios and increasing need for services that cause school counselors to increase referral activity, the academic preparation of school counselors is seriously lacking in referral training (Weinrach, 1984). According to Bobele and Conran (1988), this lack of training deters many counselors from making referrals because they are not familiar with effective procedures. In addition, referrals that are attempted are not as successful, producing many no-shows and counseling relationships that fail to thrive

(Bobele and Conran, 1988). Unsuccessful referrals are a costly waste of school resources (Zinos and Hopkins, 1981). In addition, a family that has been referred before will be less likely to accept the next referral (Conti, 1975). Therefore, it is crucial for a school counselor to be extremely skilled in connecting the family with the most appropriate counselor available.

In addition to school counselors, school psychologists spend a great deal of time referring children and their families to outside resources (Farling and Hoedt, 1971). Both school counselors and school psychologists can enhance their own effectiveness on the job by improving their referral procedures (Conti, 1975). Throughout the rest of the chapter, the word counselor will be used to refer to both school counselors and school psychologists.

Counselors are becoming more cognizant of the effectiveness of viewing the family and the school as systems. To accomplish this, the school counselor should take inventory of the available school resources, the available community resources (Downing, 1985), and the available family resources.

In taking a thorough inventory of school resources, the counselor needs to assess the school's counseling and psychology staff, their degrees, their theoretical orientation, their areas of expertise, their availability, and their interests. Next, the counselor should assess the community resources. This process is a thoroughly time-consuming one but is extremely important to the systems approach of school counseling. The assessment of community resources is covered in other chapters of this book. However, for school counselors, the issue is one of looking for community resource persons who are systems-oriented and who wish to work specifically with families in which the student is a part of a school system. Another important feature that counselors need to consider is whether the community referral resource is willing to have an ongoing relationship with the school system. Because the school system is monitoring the student's progress day by day, the school counselor will want to have reasonably ready access to the community referral resource.

According to Weinrach (1984), within five sessions the new psychologist should have a rather clear idea of the client's concerns and readiness for help. The new psychologist should commit to writing a report to the school counselor and then send an update each six-to-ten-week period if there is an impact on the student's performance in school. Weinrach agrees that this process is time-consuming but necessary to monitor the student's progress. Not every family counselor welcomes this interaction. The school counselor, therefore, needs to build a relationship with several community referral resources with whom she can have on-going dialogue concerning the student and his progress. Finally, the school counselor needs to assess the community referral resources as to their ability to meet the various needs of students and their families. For example, one counselor may specialize in defusing abusive family situations while another may specialize in helping families with a learning-disabled child. Downing (1985) states that "the degree to which a counselor is knowledgeable of local resources will largely determine the rate of success he or she will have in referring counselors."

Finally, the school counselor must assess the family's resources. Some of the family's resources include their ability to be supportive of one another, their emotional stability, their fiscal resources, their commitment to education, their physical health, their institutional support systems, and their commitment to change. The counselor should also attend to the liabilities of the family when making a referral. By assessing the family's resources or lack of resources, the community's resources, and the school system's ability to help the family, the school counselor is best able to match the needs of the family and the child (children) with the most appropriate school resources and community referral.

Earlier in this book, the topic of how to refer a client is thoroughly presented. In that presentation, the assumption is that the client is in some way known to the helper to such an extent that the helper can ask questions and explore with the client or potential client some of the necessary information that can help make the referral process succeed. However in the school setting, the first person that is brought to the counselor's attention is not the actual client but one member of a family system. The student who is identified as having the need for counseling is not the person who can commit the time and money to counseling; the actual client is the family and power to commit to counseling lies with the parents. Many times the school counselor does not even know the student's parents, and now faced with the parents for the first time has the dubious distinction of informing them that their family unit needs professional help. The questions that the counselor must ask in order to identify the family's resources and growing edges may well appear to be invasive and rude because there is no relationship on which to base the needed interaction. Therefore, the manner of making a referral must be handled very delicately at first in order to gain the family's cooperation.

Before the school counselor actually makes the referral, she must first evaluate the child's behavior and the situation that has occurred. All school staff who are involved in the decision to refer should be involved in a collaborative effort to identify the child's presenting problem behavior. After the school personnel have agreed that the child's behavior is problematic, then the family is called for a conference. Conti's research (1975) indicates that if several school personnel are involved in a referral, then the family is more likely to follow through with the referral. Therefore, it is wise to have all the school personnel who are most involved with the child attend the meeting.

PITFALLS FOR SCHOOL COUNSELORS IN REFERRALS

When presenting the referral to the family, there are several pitfalls that the counselor should avoid.

1. Do not assume that the family knows about the child's problem behavior or has observed the behavior directly.
2. Do not assume that the family understands the nature of family counseling.
3. Do not intimate that the family is crazy, wicked, and needs a shrink (Bobele and Conran, 1988). This is the surest way to alienate

the family to the helping profession and assure an unsuccessful referral.

4. Do not tell the family that the entire family has problems. simply recommend family counseling as the most appropriate means to handle the family's problem.

5. Do not set conditions such as telling the family that they must see a therapist or else . . . Setting conditions will make the family therapist's job more difficult because the family may feel manipulated into counseling and will therefore be resistant from the first appointment, if they follow through at all. The arm twisting may have to occur later if the family does not voluntarily seek help for the problem, but initially the meeting should have the ambience of a cooperative search for provision of optimal resources for the family.

6. Do not oversimplify the problem by telling the family that the problem is easily corrected. If the problem was a simple one, then the family would have found a way to solve it themselves.

7. Do not tell the family that counseling is their last resort. Usually this is not true because there are always alternatives to pursue.

8. Avoid setting fees or making other promises on behalf of the family therapist.

9. Do not disguise the therapist as a consultant or other helping professional. Being honest with the family will gain respect for the entire mental health system (Bobele and Conran, 1988).

10. Do not make specific promises about counseling outcome or procedure, or about medication.

SCHOOL COUNSELORS AND REFERRALS THAT WORK

The school counselor must be well prepared for the meeting with the family.

1. School counselors will have more success with referral if they describe the behavior of the child instead of offering impressions,

thoughts, and feelings. Families are more likely to respond to the counselor's suggestion for referral if they are presented with concrete behavior that is described clearly, succinctly, and with appropriate examples. The school counselor must therefore be prepared for the meeting with the family.

2. At the family and school personnel conference, provide enough time to thoroughly discuss the referral (Downing, 1985). Communicate confidence in the therapist and in the family's ability to succeed.

3. Explain the concept of family counseling enough to make them comfortable without overexplaining. Let the family therapist explain all the details, rules, and boundaries of family counseling.

4. Let the family take the initiative in contacting the family counselor. Give the family the specific names, addresses, and telephone numbers of professionals and/or specific agencies who can best serve the family. Some school counselors even offer their telephone to the family so that the appointment can be initiated at the moment of commitment.

5. At the conference with the family, focus on the needs of the family and the connection of those needs with family counseling services.

6. Obtain a release of confidential information from the family with the understanding that information will not be forwarded until the family therapist asks for the school records.

7. Request permission to contact the family and family therapist in a few weeks to see whether the family is receiving the help that is required. This follow-through shows interest and encouragement and also allows the counselor to evaluate the effectiveness of the referral process and the new therapeutic relationship (Downing, 1985; Conti, 1975). For further information, on follow-up, see other sections of this book.

CONCLUSION

School counselors and school psychologists need excellent referral skills due to the extremely high student-counselor ratios that are currently the norm in school systems. Counselors who approach referral as an extremely sensitive, interactive, and difficult process are capable of making successful referrals to family therapists and other mental health professionals. Counselors who see referral as an innocuous procedure that allows them to slough families onto other counselors with little thought or follow-through will make referrals that frequently fail to meet families' needs (Weinrach, 1984). Since the research shows that families who are receiving second or third referrals are unlikely to follow through on the referral appointment, it is incumbent on all school counselors to take the additional time and effort to assure that the first referral is well-conceived and appropriate to the family's needs (Conti, 1975).

13

Referral Practices in Parish Ministry

When a person is in physical pain, the first professional who is contacted is usually a physician. When a person is in psychic pain, the first professional who is contacted is usually an ordained minister (King, 1978). Yet according to research, the referral rate for ministers is extremely low (Gilbert, 1981; Worthington, 1986; Bell et al., 1976). In addition, ministers rarely receive a referral from a mental health professional (Bell et al., 1976; Cummings and Harrington, 1963). The interaction between clergy and mental health professionals is limited. Considering the significant number of people turning to ministers during their time of need and a concomitant low referral rate from ministers to mental health professionals, either clergy must be performing a great deal of counseling or else, even though clients contact their pastor, clients must actually be receiving their referrals from sources other than their pastors. A third alternative may exist. That is, ministers see clients for a period of time, clients feel somewhat better and are therefore not in as much need of an immediate referral, so none is made.

WHY PASTORS ARE RELUCTANT TO REFER

Perhaps the clue to the dilemma rests with the reasons pastors are reluctant to refer their parishioners and others who come to see them for counseling. In researching the referral practices of ministers, Lowe (1986) found that ministers feel the need to be more adequately trained in counseling in order to handle situations themselves. Lowe also found that they were least interested in entering the referral system. This research and other supporting data (Oglesby, 1978; Gilbert, 1981) indicates the autonomy that pastors in general feel about their counseling duties. The implications are serious and need to be addressed by an interaction between pastors and mental health professionals. Lowe (1986) raises an ethical concern about nonreferring pastors who have limited amounts of formal counseling training. Problems seen by clergy appear to be equal in magnitude to those seen generally be mental health professionals. Yet mental health professionals spend years in training in order to learn the myriad skills necessary to work with the variety of mental health concerns. Even with extensive training, mental health practitioners refer cases which are beyond their capabilities to other professionals. However, from the research presented in the journals, pastors are reluctant to refer.

In his research, Worthington (1986) attempted to understand the nonreferral activity of many pastors. He found that pastors preferred to know the religious orientation of the therapists to whom they referred clients. Gilbert's (1981a) research supported Worthington's outcome in that referral by pastors was most strongly affected by their theological orientation. Theologically conservative clergy were more likely to be isolated from mental health professionals while theologically liberal clergy were more likely to refer to mental health professionals. However, conservative or liberal, clergy expressed dissatisfaction with available counseling services and expressed concern that the client's (parishioner's) faith would be misunderstood, unappreciated, or even ridiculed by an agnostic or atheistic counselor (King, 1978). Indeed, some mental health professionals view religion or faith as one symptom of psychopathology. Is it any wonder then, that clergy are hesitant to refer to mental health professionals? Gilbert (1981a) found that this hesitancy is especially true of clergy who are authoritarian or who have a poor self-concept. In addition, pastors of small churches were less likely to refer than were pastors of large churches (500 or more members). Pastors, however, who were highly educated, who had high counseling activity, and who regularly interacted with a variety of professional colleagues were more likely to refer clients to a mental health facility (Rumberger and Rogers, 1987).

Clinebell (1966) asserts a different reason for the nonreferral behavior of clergy. He contends that pastors are seen by their congregations as representing God and if, for any reason, the pastor should refer a parishioner outside the church, then the pastor, the church, and God may be perceived as having failed that person. Oglesby (1978) supports Clinebell's assertion, but further suggests that clergy overvalue their own resources and devalue any resources that are not a part of the church.

Finally, clergy are sensitive to parishioners' feelings of rejection. Pastors want their parishioners to feel welcome at the church and to feel that the church community can meet their needs. Referral outside that community is seen as an admission of the church's inability to meet its members' needs.

CHALLENGING THE MYTH OF THE CLERGY-MENTAL HEALTH SCHISM

The Pastoral Challenge

Pastor's mistrust of human service professionals is grounded in an historical and philosophical difference of opinion over the nature of humankind. Earlier psychological theorists saw people as determined by their unconscious, and scoffed at religious faith as magical thinking and pathological dependency. The primary orientation of church leaders is more existential, emphasizing freedom and responsibility. The scientists of psychology and psychiatry appreciate concrete data while pastors rely on faith and intuition. While these polarities do still exist, there is a trend toward a more holistic, multidisciplinary approach to assisting clients. Human service professionals are beginning to respect the contributions of all fields. In fact, the entire field of pastoral counseling has developed in the last twenty years, in which the integration of psychology and spirituality is the major goal. While research shows that 95 percent of psychologists and 57 percent of psychiatrists do not believe in God (Larson, 1986), through simple subtraction it is evident that 5 percent of psychologists and 43 percent of psychiatrists *do* believe in God. Therefore, ordained clergy need not avoid the mental health professions but should identify and interact with those practitioners who share a similar faith experience. The first obvious source of referral possibilities is the pastor's own congregation. The second place where clergy may find referral resources is through other clergy who may know of mental health professionals in their congregations. Finally clergy interact in a number of community settings where mental health professionals also are involved. Pastors can build their contacts in hospital settings, hospice settings, police departments, fire departments, and social service settings. Finally, Oglesby (1978) recommends that pastors look to the major professional organizations because each organization has a division or subdivision that addresses the concerns of professionals who want to integrate psychology and theology. Lists are available of members who choose to belong to these divisions.

The Mental Health Professional Challenge

Mental health professionals must bear some of the responsibility for the lack of interaction between themselves and clergy. There is a tradition for mental health professionals to view clergy as outside the mental health field or as only interested in a person's relationship to God. This view is antiquated and needs revision. Most clergy are concerned with the whole person and his or her community: interpersonal relationships, intrapersonal relationship, the person's relationship to God, the person's view of life, grief issues, physical health, and emotional health. Pastors are also frequently concerned with issues of peace, justice, education (secular and religious), the environment, social problems, and politics. Mental health professionals who are unaware of the contribution of clergy to the well-being of their parishioners and the community are missing valuable allies. Clients value their pastor's input and advice. This is well-documented in the literature (King, 1978; Gilbert, 1981; Worthington, 1986). Mental health professionals need to see the value of pastors' contributions to the mental health field and the value of the pastor as a colleague in assisting with the health of clients.

Contact between the two professionals can be initiated by either party, but mental health professionals who treat pastors as colleagues will find a valuable resource as well as referral potential on both sides. Not only will clients be referred from the pastors to the mental health professional, but also, clients can be referred to pastors for spiritual direction or access to various community resources. In addition, some pastors hold additional advanced degrees in counseling and psychotherapy and are, therefore, as well trained as mental health professionals. These pastors should be viewed as any other competent counselor with a plus—their pastoral identity.

CHALLENGING THE MYTH THAT REFERRAL OUTSIDE THE CHURCH IS FAILURE

Pastors who attempt to handle practically all of the counseling required by their congregations and who rarely utilize referral as a therapeutic intervention are similar to counselors who attempt to treat all clients who present themselves for counseling. They fear that referral means failure. Oglesby (1978) contends that this activity is most prevalent among clergy who believe that the Gospel should be adequate to solve all problems and that referral is an admission that the Gospel is inadequate. Some ministers do not place as much healing emphasis on the Gospel but contend that the church community should be sufficient to solve relationship problems or that to refer is an admission that they, as pastors, are incapable of helping the very people whom they were called to serve. However, the Gospel does cite situations in which God models the utilization of others as instruments of healing. God works through many channels, most of which we scarcely understand. In Luke, John brought to Jesus's attention a man who was casting out demons in Christ's name. John asked Jesus to forbid the man from casting out demons, but Jesus said, "Do not forbid him; for he that is not against you is for you." Oglesby states "The power of God is not limited to those channels which overtly attest to His presence, nor is healing any less a matter of faith even though certain theological symbols are not in evidence."

Pastors need to see themselves as a valuable part of a community in which there is continuous interaction between all community and church resources. Instead of viewing referral as a failure to provide needed services, pastors need to see referral as a powerful helping tool that enriches the resources of the church and brings the healthy resources of the community to the church. A pastor can still be mindful of referring a parishioner to a counselor whose religious values and world views match the church's and, most importantly, the client's.

CHALLENGING THE MYTH THAT CLERGY OVERVALUE THEIR OWN RESOURCES AND UNDERVALUE THE RESOURCES OF MENTAL HEALTH PROFESSIONALS

Clergy may choose to avoid referral because they overvalue the type and amount of help that they can give to parishioners and devalue the gifts of the secular world. However, the assumption that there is a rigid split between the sacred and secular worlds is erroneous. The very parishioners who sit in church are the ones who then leave church to work in the secular world. If religious faith is to work in the world, then the parishioners must enter the world to practice that faith. The church through the work of its members ought to be impacting the secular community, not remaining detached from it. The physician who goes to church to profess his faith is still the same person who enters the office on Monday to practice his skills. Pastors must not avoid referral, but only search out which referral source is the most commensurate with the client's needs, including his faith needs.

The pastor who decides to counsel all those in need with little regard for the community resources, is overvaluing her skills. This is especially true of pastors who have little training in counseling. Gilbert (1981) found in his research that the least trained pastors were doing proportionately more counseling than the more highly trained pastors. The implication is that parishioners who need professional mental health intervention may not be receiving it due to passive or even active resistance to referral by their pastors.

While almost all pastors do some counseling, each pastor must assess her own abilities honestly, learn how and when to refer to others, and obtain additional training in counseling if interested in routinely providing ongoing counseling services to parishioners. The last suggestion is probably the most appropriate answer for pastors who wish to handle most counseling needs within the auspices of the church. Additional counseling training would sharpen the clergy person's diagnostic skills, increase the scope of her intervention strategies, and allow her to develop a sense of her own abilities and growing edges.

CHALLENGING THE MYTH THAT PARISHIONERS FEEL REJECTION UPON REFERRAL

Pastors who are reluctant to refer because of a fear that parishioners will feel rejected are referred to other sections of this book where a discussion of client rejection and referral is given. However, the pastor presents a slightly unique situation with regard to referral and rejection. Since counseling parishioners is seen as a part of a minister's duties, a parishioner may have difficulty in understanding why the pastor is referring him while continuing to see others in an ongoing counseling relationship. Traditionally, the pastor is nor allowed to say that she has no additional time for counseling parishioners because in most churches the minister is to be on call and available for the congregation twenty-four hours a day. Some members of the congregation may even believe that through their weekly offering they have purchased the pastor's time and availability. In contrast, the client who has been referred to another counselor must purchase the services. In the pastor's case, the parishioner may feel that he has already purchased the service and has paid for it over many years and now he wishes to take advantage of his option.

It is at this point that clergy needs to set some boundaries around their role. First, a pastor must make clear to the congregation the difference between pastoral care and (pastoral) counseling. Second, a pastor needs to clarify where her skills lie and what her limitations are. Third, the pastor must discriminate between crisis intervention and ongoing therapy. Fourth, the pastor should decide approximately how many hours a week she can dedicate to ongoing counseling, if she it trained to provide this. Finally, the pastor should educate the congregation on the pastor's important role of referral.

The wise pastor makes the above information available and overt from the minute she enters the life of the congregation. In this way, parishioners are not surprised if the pastor must refer. In fact, the pastor may have parishioners enter her office for the purpose of receiving a referral. Pastors whose judgment is respected by their congregation will find that a well-conceived referral to an appropriate counselor is an important act of pastoral care. Not only will such clarification and boundary-setting enable the pastor to make referrals when needed without the parishioners' feeling rejected, but it also will model healthy boundary setting for the congregation.

Another way that a pastoral referral often differs from a purely mental health referral is that the pastor will continue to have an ongoing relationship with the client/parishioner after the referral is made. Because the pastor will continue to be involved and interested in the parishioner's problems, the parishioner may not feel as rejected as the pastor many fear. In fact, the pastor should assure the parishioner that she intends to remain involved by offering pastoral care. Therefore, the pastor is in a perfect situation to follow-up on the referral as a form of her pastoral care. Even though the referral was made to a mental health professional, the pastor may still be involved with a person's crisis or grief. It is therefore critical that the lines of communication be open between the referral resource and the pastor whenever the client is utilizing the services of both the counselor and pastor. This will eliminate the possibility of the pastor and the counselor working against each other inadvertently. Of course, the necessary release-of-confidential-information form must be signed (see Appendix A).

TO COUNSEL OR NOT TO COUNSEL MEMBERS OF THE PASTOR'S CONGREGATION

Pastors see counseling as a part of their normal duties within the church setting. For most pastors, counseling consists of crises management, marital counseling, grief counseling, pre-marital counseling, and spiritual direction. Ongoing therapeutic work is usually left to mental health practitioners. However, when a pastor has studied counseling at the graduate level, the pastor begins to act as a mental health professional and is able to enter long-term therapeutic relationships. When this occurs, some pastors have found that a conflict of interest can develop from the dual relationship. When practicing intensive psychotherapy, transference is encouraged, insight is obtained, resistance is often seen, and confrontation is often needed. The conflicts, anger, and attempt at manipulative behavior that occur are a normal part of this long-term process where a person is attempting to reconstruct his personality. If this person is also a parishioner and interacts with the pastor, who is also his therapist, on day-to-day activities in the parish, then the conflicts, anger, resistance, and manipulation can ooze out of the therapeutic sessions and contaminate the parish activities.

Pastors who experience this type of dual relationship are often apt to refer all parishioners who need long-term counseling to other trained therapists. Other pastors report that they are extremely successful in maintaining the boundaries and using the contamination activities of the client as learning experiences. Lay persons working as pastoral counselors in their own parishes have similar experiences. The difficulty is one of boundaries. Pastors who find the dual relationship nontherapeutic will find it beneficial to have reciprocal referral relationships with other therapeutically trained pastors and mental health professionals. Pastors who are able to work within the dual structure must establish sacred boundaries with their clients/parishioners and be ever mindful of the possibility that a referral may become necessary.

In a previous chapter, the subject of lack of referral resources was discussed as one problem that counselors need to address. Pastors who serve small parishes in rural areas are faced with the problem of few if any referral resources. When this happens, pastors are forced to enter counseling relationships with those parish members and community members who have no other recourse. However, Gilbert (1981) suggests that many pastors in rural settings are unaware or misinformed regarding the availability of mental health professionals in their area. (see section on building referrals in rural settings). Pastors who are in isolated areas and have no referral resources but feel the obligation to do counseling should consider the following suggestions to bring more quality into their counseling activities:

1. Seek supervision even if you must drive a long distance. If no supervision is available, then seek some type of consultation.
2. Attend a graduate school program in counseling or at least schedule time to travel for seminar and workshops to improve your skills.
3. Encourage a local resident who seems interested in what you are doing to become trained in counseling, even if it is paraprofessional counseling training or peer counseling.
4. Organize a group of lay men and women who appear to be good listeners to form a reach-out group ministry and help them use

each other and you as consultants. The sharing can generate excellent consultation.

5. Join a behavioral science book club and immerse yourself in reading about counseling strategies.

6. Continue to look for referral possibilities.

APPENDIX A

Sample Forms

REFERRAL RESOURCE DATA BASE

BASIC INFORMATION

Entry Date: ___________

PERSONAL

Title: ____
First Name: ________________ Last Name: ______________________
Address: ____
City: ______________________ State: _____ Zip: ____________ DOB: _______
Home Phone: ______________________________________ Sex: _______

PROFESSIONAL

Place of Work: ______________________________________
Work Address: ______________________________________
City: ______________________ State: _____ Zip: ____________
Work Phone: ____
Profession: ________________ Areas of Expertise: ______________________
____

ADDITIONAL INFORMATION

Recommending Counselor: ______________________________

Referral Resource:	Y ___	N ___
Referral Source:	Y ___	N ___
Client:	Y ___	N ___
Personal Friend:	Y ___	N ___
Ever Made a Referral to Agency:	Y ___	N ___

Religious Affiliation: ______________________________
Comments: ____
____

COUNSELING REFERRAL FORM
TYPE A

LOGO

Dear ____________________________________,

The following names are being provided to you by ________________________ (therapist) for the purpose of referral. Please feel free to contact any of these referral resources directly as each has been notified to expect your call. If for any reason you are not comfortable with those listed below, please contact me for the names of additional professionals. Have new professional send signed release of confidential information to me as appropriate to request information.

Name:

Address:

Phone:

Name:

Address:

Phone:

Name:

Address:

Phone:

Sincerely,

______________________________ (Therapist)

______________________________ (Address)

____

______________________________ (Phone)

Please use my name when contacting the new profressional.

COUNSELING REFERRAL FORM
TYPE B

LOGO

To ______________________________ (Client)

From ______________________________ (Therapist)

Date ______________________________

Re: Referral

The following referral resources are being provided to you. Please follow instructions on the bottom of this form.

#1 Name:

Address:

Phone:

#2 Name:

Address:

Phone:

#3 Name:

Address:

Phone:

☐ Contact helper of your choice

☐ Counselor # ______ will be calling you. If this referral is not satisfactory, please feel free to contact either of the other two professionals or myself for additional referral resources.

Please use my name when contacting the new therapist. Have new therapist send signed release of confidential information to me as appropriate to obtain information.

RELEASE OF CONFIDENTIAL INFORMATION FORM

(PASTE IN)

APPENDIX

B

National Organizations and Local Resources

NATIONAL ORGANIZATIONS

American Psychiatric Association
1400 K Street NW
Washington, DC 20009
National referrals: (202) 682-6121

American Psychiatrist Biographical Directory
R. R. Bowker Publications
P. O. Box 1807
Ann Arbor, Michigan 48106

American Psychological Association
1200 17th Street NW
Washington, DC 20036
(202) 955-7600

American Association of Pastoral Counselors
9508A Lee Highway
Fairfax, Virginia 22031
(703) 385-6967

American Association for Counseling and Development
5999 Stevenson Lane
Alexandria, Virginia 22304
(703) 823-9800
(800) 545-AACD

National Board for Certified Counselors
Suite 402
5999 Stevenson Avenue
Alexandria, Virginia 22304
(703) 461-NBCC

American Association of Marriage and Family Therapists
Registry of Service Providers
225 Yale Avenue
Claremont, California 91711

National Association of Social Workers
7981 Eastern Avenue
Silver Spring, Maryland 20910
(301) 565-0333

Family Service Association of America
(A national accrediting, standards-setting organization of 300 nonprofit volunteer family social services)
Directory of Member Agencies
44 E. 23rd Street
New York, New York 10010

National Association for Retarded Citizens
2709 Avenue East
P.O. Box 6109
Arlington, Texas 76011

National Academy of Certified Clinical Mental Health Counselors
5999 Stevenson Lane
Alexandria, Virginia 22304
(703) 823-9800

LOCAL RESOURCES (SEE LOCAL TELEPHONE DIRECTORY)

Child Guidance Clinics at local hospitals or medical schools

Psychiatric Outpatient Clinics (call local United Way)

Community Mental Health Centers

Alcoholics Anonymous
(national; for local AA see telephone directory)
P.O. Box 459, Grand Central Station
New York, New York 10017

Planned Parenthood (national; for local see telephone directory)
810 7th Avenue
New York, New York 10019
(212) 541-7800

American Red Cross
emergency disability for military families; AIDS testing

Catholic Charities
National Conference of Catholic Charities
1346 Connecticut Avenue NW
Washington, DC 20036

Jewish Health and Welfare Agencies
Council of Jewish Federations
575 Lexington Avenue
New York, New York 10022

Rescue Missions—rooms and lodging
Salvation Army (national; for local see telephone directory)
120 West 14th Street
New York, New York 10011

Private Practice Institute
581 Forest Avenue
Portland, Maine 04101
(800) 338-3748

*References and Selected Bibliography**

➡ Abramczyk, L. W. (1981). The counseling function of pastors: A study in practice and preparation. *Journal of Psychology and Theology, 9,* 257–265.

American Association for Counseling and Development Ethical Standards. (1988). Springfield: AACD.

➡ American Psychiatric Association Task Force Report 10: Psychiatrists' viewpoints on religion and their services to religious institutions and the ministry. (1975). Washington, DC: American Psychiatric Association.

Bell, R. A., Morris, R. R., Holzer, C. E., and Warheit, G. J. (1976). The clergy as a mental health resource: Parts I and II. *The Journal of Pastoral Care, 30,* 103–115.

Bobele, M., and Conran, T. J. (1988). Referral for family therapy: Pitfalls and guidelines. *Elementary School Counseling, 22,* 192–198.

Cavanaugh, M. E. (1980). Becoming a more effective helper. Keynote speech, 25th Anniversary of McAuley Neuropsychiatric Institute, San Francisco.

* References marked with an arrow do not appear in the text, but were used by the author in preparation of this book.

Clinebell, H. (1966). *Basic types of pastoral counseling.* Nashville: Abingdon Press.

Conti, A. P. (1975). Variables related to contacting/ not contacting counseling services recommended by school psychologists. *Journal of School Psychology, 13,* 41–50.

➥ Cornell, W. (1988). Maintaining an independent private practice: An opinion. *The Script,* Jan.–Feb., 1988.

Cummings, E., and Harrington, C. (1969). Clergymen and Counseling. American Journal of Sociology, 234–243.

Downing, C. J. (1985). Referrals that work. *The School Counselor, 32,* 242–246.

Farling, W., and Hoedt, K. (1971). National Survey of School Psychology. U.S. Dept. of Health, Education and Welfare, Washington, D.C.

Garfield, S. L. (1980). *Psychotherapy: An eclectic approach.* New York: Wiley.

Gilbert, M. G. (1981). The decision of Assemblies of God pastors to counsel or refer. *Journal of Psychology and Theology, 9,* 250–256.

——— (1981a). Characteristics of pastors related to pastoral counseling and referral. *Journal of Pastoral Counseling, 16,* 30–38.

Gould, R. L., Paulson, I., and Daniels-Epps, L. (1970). Patients who flirt with treatment: The silent population. *American Journal of Psychiatry, 127,* 524–529.

➥ Gouvier, D., Webster, J. and Blanton, P. (1986). Cognitive retraining with brain damaged patients. *The Neurophychology Handbook.* New York: Springer, 278–324.

➥ Hong, B. A., and Wine, V. R. (1975). Referral patterns of clergy. *Journal of Psychology and Theology, 3,* 291–297.

Hopkins, B., and Anderson, B. (1985). The Counselor and the Law (2nd ed.) Springfield: American Association for Counseling and Development.

➥ Horton, A. and Sautter, S. (1986). Behavioral neuropsychology: Behavioral treatment for brain injured. *The Neuropsychology Handbook.* New York: Springer, 259–277.

King, R. R. (1978). Evangelical Christians and professional counseling: A conflict of values. *Journal of Psychology and Theology, 6,* 276–281.

Larson, et al. (1986). Systematic analysis of research on religious variables in four major psychiatric journals, 1978–1982. *American Journal of Psychiatry, 143,* 329–334.

➥ Lewis, L. (1986). Individual psychotherapy with patients have combined psychological and neurological disorders. *Bulletin of Menninger Clinic, 50,* 75–87.

Lewis, L., and Swiercinski, D. (1981). Consideration in referring patients for neuropsychological assessment. *Bulletin of the Menninger Clinic, 45,* 442–446.

➥ Lezak, M. D. (1983). *Neuropsychological Assessment* (2nd ed.). New York: Oxford University Press.

Lowe, D. W. (1986). Counseling activities and referral practices of ministers. *Journal of Psychology and Christianity, 5,* 22–29.

➥ Margenau, E. (ed.). (1990). *Encyclopedic Handbook of Private Practice.* New York: Gardner Press, Inc.

Miach, A., Elliott, J., and Cava, J. (1979). The referring therapist's expectations of inpatient treatment. *Canadian Journal of Psychiatry, 24,* 749–754.

Oglesby, W. B. Jr. (1978). *Referral in pastoral counseling.* Nashville: Abingdon Press.

➥ O'Neil, J. M., Price, G. E., and Eads, D. (1978). An empirical investigation of the counseling referral process. *Journal of College Student Personnel,* July, 306–308.

➥ Paul, G. L. (1967). Strategy of outcome research in psychotherapy. *Journal of Consulting Psychology, 31,* 109–118.

➥ Piedmont, E. B. (1969). Referrals and reciprocity: psychiatrists, general practitioners and clergymen. *Journal of Health and Social Behavior,* 29–41.

Raynes, A. E., and Warren, G., (1971). Some distinguishing features of patients failing to attend a psychiatric clinic after referral. *American Journal of Orthopsychiatry, 41,* 581–588.

Ritchie, M. H. (1988). Ethical procedures for referral and termination. Paper presented at Association for Counselor Education and Supervision National Conference, October 9, 1988.

➥ Rogers, C. (1961). *On becoming a person.* Boston: Houghton Mifflin.

➥ Rosenthal, M. and Geckler, C. (1976). Family Therapy Issues in neuropsychology. The Neuropsychology Handbook. New York: Springer, 325–346.

Rumberger, O. J., and Rogers, M. L. (1987). Pastoral openness to interact with private Christian counseling services. *Journal of Psychology and Theology, 10,* 337–345.

Shullman, S. and Betz, N. (1979). An investigation of the effects of client sex and presenting problem in referral from intake. *Journal of Counseling Psychology, 26,* 140–145.

➥ Virkler, H. A. (1979). Counseling demands, procedures and preparations of parish ministers: A descriptive study. *Journal of Psychology and Theology, 7,* 271–280.

Weinrach, S. A. (1984). Toward improved referral making: Mutuality between the counselor and the psychologist. *The School Counselor, 31,* 89–96.

➥ Weiss, R. S. (1973). Helping relationships of clients with physicians, social workers, priests and others. *Social Problems, 20,* 319–328.

Worthington, E. L. Jr. (1986). Religious counseling: A review of published empirical research. *Journal of Counseling and Development, 64,* 421–431.

Zinos, J. E., and Hopkins, R. A. (1981). Referrals out: Increasing the numbers of kept appointments. *School Psychology Review, 10,* 107–111.

Index

SHARON E. CHESTON

Dr. Cheston is an associate chair of the Pastoral Counseling Department at Loyola College in Maryland. As a counselor educator and supervisor, Dr. Cheston has been teaching and supervising novice and experienced counselors in the art of helping since 1986. Dr. Cheston's interest in the subject of therapeutic referral is born out of her extensive experience in aiding therapists in assessing their own strengths while determining their clients' needs for appropriate types of therapy.

Dr. Cheston is a National Certified Counselor, a National Certified Mental Health Counselor, and a Certified Professional Counselor in the state of Maryland. In addition to her position at Loyola College, Dr. Cheston has a private practice with Bay Ridge Counseling Center, Inc. and resides in a suburb of Baltimore with her family.